Intermittent Fasting for Women Over 50

2021

The Ultimate Guide to Quickk Weight Loss

© **Copyright 2021 - All rights reserved.**

This document is geared towards providing exact and reliable information in regards to the topic and issue covered. The publication is sold with the idea that the publisher is not required to render accounting, officially permitted, or otherwise, qualified services. If advice is necessary, legal or professional, a practiced individual in the profession should be ordered.

- From a Declaration of Principles which was accepted and approved equally by a Committee of the American Bar Association and a Committee of Publishers and Associations.

In no way is it legal to reproduce, duplicate, or transmit any part of this document in either electronic means or in printed format. Recording of this publication is strictly prohibited, and any storage of this document is not allowed unless with written permission from the publisher. All rights reserved.

The information provided herein is stated to be truthful and consistent, in that any liability, in terms of inattention or otherwise, by any usage or abuse of any policies, processes, or Instructions contained within is the solitary and utter responsibility of the recipient reader. Under no circumstances will any legal responsibility or blame be held against the publisher for any reparation, damages, or monetary loss due to the information herein, either directly or indirectly.

Respective authors own all copyrights not held by the publisher.

The information herein is offered for informational purposes solely and is universal as such. The presentation of the information is without a contract or any type of guarantee assurance.

The trademarks that are used are without any consent, and the publication of the trademark is without permission or backing by the trademark owner. All trademarks and brands within this book are for clarifying purposes only and are owned by the owners themselves, not affiliated with this document.

Table of Contents

Introduction

Chapter 1: Basics of Concept of Fasting

Chapter 2: Should IF be Adapted?

   2.1 Is Intermittent Fasting Worth It?

Chapter 3: Types Of Intermittent Fasting

   3.1 Which Kind Of Intermittent Fasting Is Best For You?

   3.2 Protocols Of Intermittent Fasting

Chapter 4: How Does Intermittent Fasting Work?

   4.1 The Process Behind IF

   4.2 Short Fasting Regimens – Less Than 24 Hours

   4.3 Different Durations

   4.4 Short Regimens 12-Hour Fasting

   4.5 16-Hour Fasting

   4.6 What's The Point Of Incorporating Daily Fasting?

   4.7 Alternate Daily Fasting (ADF)

   4.8 Complications Risk Of Fasts >24 Hours

Chapter 5: Intermittent Fasting For Women After 50

   5.1 Key Benefits Of Intermittent Fasting For Over 50 Women

   5.2 Women Over 50 May Extend Beyond Calorie Restriction

   5.3 Typical Results Of Intermittent Fasting

   5.4 Intermittent Fasting As Best Fat-Loss Tool

Chapter 6: Considering Factors Before Trying IF

Chapter 7: What Intermittent Fasting Does and Doesn't Do?

   7.1 Burning Stored Fat

   7.2 Intermittent Fasting Is Not For Everyone

   7.3 What Exactly Is The Purpose Of Fasting?

   7.4 Is Intermittent Fasting Right For You?

   7.5 How To Shape Up Without Intermittent Fasting?

Chapter 8: Health Benefits of Intermittent Fasting

Chapter 9: Best Foods During Intermittent Fasting

Chapter 10: Foods to Avoid while Intermittent Fasting

Chapter 11: Must Avoiding Mistakes While Intermittent Fasting

Chapter 12: Intermittent Fasting Tips For Success

Chapter 13: Healthy Recipes For Intermittent Faster

13.1 Best Food To Break An Intermittent Fast

13.2 Delicious and Healthy Recipes

Conclusion

Introduction

Thanks for choosing this book, make sure to leave a short review on Amazon if you enjoy it, I'd really love to hear your thoughts.

You may have come across the phrase "Intermittent Fasting" from time to time. Despite how frightening the term may seem, this strategy is simple to implement. In addition, it was named the most popular weight-loss approach in 2019. If you've tried fasting before, you'll find that intermittent fasting isn't difficult to follow. It's also not required to be acquainted with the notion of fasting to practice intermittent fasting. Intermittent fasting has gained popularity all around the world, and many individuals practice it daily. It offers a lot more advantages than you may realize.

'What is intermittent fasting,' you may be wondering. In the long term, intermittent fasting involves energy restriction regularly. It's a timed cycle of daily meal preparation that alternates between fasting and non-fasting periods. You eat just two meals each day and then fast for 16 hours before eating again. Yes, you may wonder why just two meals are served; but, as we go through the book.

It is not required for everyone to fast for 16 hours; some individuals lack the energy to do so perfectly. You may also break down regular fasting strategies by fasting for just a shorter period while remembering to consume two meals per day that adequately satisfy your hunger. You may dine between the hours of 9 a.m. and 5 p.m. or between 1 p.m. and 8 p.m. You've got 6-7 hours to eat on your own. However, don't go overboard with your food consumption. You're still on a diet, so keep that in mind.

Intermittent fasting (IF) is one of the most popular fitness and health fads globally.

People are using it to help them lose weight, improve their health, and simplify their lives.

Many studies have shown that it may have a significant impact on your body and brain and may even increase longevity.

Intermittent fasting is eating that alternates between fasting and eating sessions. It doesn't tell you which meals to consume, but rather when you will consume them. In this way, it's more correctly defined as an eating habit rather than a diet in the traditional sense.

Fasting for 16 hours twice a week or 24 hours once a week are two common intermittent fasting approaches.

Fasting has been a part of human culture since the beginning of time. Grocery stores, refrigerators, and year-round food were not accessible to ancient hunter-gatherers. They sometimes went hungry since they couldn't find anything to eat.

As a consequence, humans have developed to be able to survive for long periods without eating.

Fasting is, in fact, more natural than eating 3–4 or maybe more meals each day regularly.

Fasting is often practiced in Islam, Christianity, Judaism, and Buddhism for religious or spiritual reasons.

Intermittent fasting is eating that alternates between fasting and eating intervals. In the fitness and health sector, it's highly trendy right now.

Chapter 1: Basics of Concept of Fasting

Fasting is a period in which you refrain from consuming food. Before you begin a fast, the following are guidelines of interest to medical professionals

Intermittent fasting is in the limelight more these days because of the popularity of fasting and the number of loud advocates it has, which are especially notable for the amount of weight reduction, heart health, and lifespan it may help produce. To find out what precisely fasting is and whether it deserves all the praise and health claims, one must undertake it.

As one research group in a 2018 BMC Complementary & Alternative Medicine study described it, fasting is "the purposeful abstention of some or all caloric meals or drinks for medicinal, spiritual, or political reasons." Most forms of fasting have the same goal in mind: to restrict what you can and cannot eat or restrict when you can and cannot eat. Although each category of fast has unique lists of benefits and risks, it is crucial to consider your overall health and goals before implementing a fast to make proven to be the best fit for you.

Fasting is very old

Most importantly, intermittent fasting is just as ancient as time, as is documented in Mark Mattson, adjunct professor of neurology at Johns Hopkins University, who states, "It goes back to the dawn of time." The whole story is rather simple: our forefathers, according to him, would eat because there was food and fasting when there wasn't. Our organ systems developed so that they work effectively while receiving irregular feeds, explains Mattson. These individuals starved when food was scarce because they were not able to function. These individuals failed to reproduce because they were unable to perform when food was limited. The survival of the fittest was the key to success.

Fasting isn't only for weight

There are many different reasons for fasting, including weight reduction and long-term health maintenance. Hunger strikes have historically been used as a method of nonviolent protest to draw attention to perceived injustices committed by a government, for example. After the death of Mahatma Gandhi in 1948, his eldest son, Hari, began a 16-month hunger strike, repeating his father's tactics against British authority.

Religious observances

In some religions, periods of fasting are encouraged. Muslim participants are supposed to refrain from food and drink for 30 days of Ramadan, and this is done to keep them focused on those who are less fortunate and underline the importance of thankfulness. On Yom Kippur, the Jewish religion requires participants to spend a day of atonement by refraining from eating and drinking from sunset until dark on the following evening. Most of the fasting that Greek Orthodox Christians practice involves giving up meat for certain periods, notably the 40 days around Christmas, the three weeks surrounding Easter, and the eight days around the Theotokos's (the Mother of God) Assumption. Mormons, also known as church members of Jesus Christ of Those last Saints, often fast on one Sunday every month for some time from 12 to 24 hours. These religious traditions serve as templates for various dry fasting techniques.

Surgery prep

To get ready for surgery, you must also go without food or water. You will be requested to refrain from eating or drinking for a certain period before an operation, such as surgery or any form of treatment that requires the use of an anesthetic. To keep nausea at bay and prevent food or fluids from going into the lungs, this is done. If you are fasting before surgery, follow your surgeon's exact instructions on when to avoid eating or drinking, plus understand exactly the regulations for drinking water during fasting if you are set for surgery.

Chapter 2: Should IF be Adapted?

Intermittent fasting is a form of diet plan in which you switch between eating and fasting on a daily basis. Intermittent fasting has been shown in studies to help people lose weight & prevent — or even cure — illness. So how do you go about doing it? Is it also safe?

Many diets emphasis what to consume, but intermittent fasting focuses when to eat.

Intermittent fasting (IF) which is a lifestyle that involves cycling among periods of eating & periods of fasting, which you will already realize if you track balanced eating and weight loss patterns. The premise being that through limiting what you feed, you will regulate the amount of calories you consume and, ideally, reap the hormonal and cellular advantages of fasting, such as lower cholesterol, improved cardiac wellbeing, and, eventually, longer life. These arguments are founded on research into the impact of IF on various markers, but they do not say the whole story. The impact of intermittent fasting on longevity & wellbeing, and so spent a lot of time trying to figure out how much IF will influence our health.

Fasting has been practiced for centuries in a multitude of societies and communities for ritual, social, educational, and political purposes. Intermittent fasting, on the other hand, is a form of calorie restriction that essentially entails eating for a span of time but then not eating for another. Since there is no one-size-fits-all approach to IF, it usually involves limiting food consumption in one of two ways: time-restricted diet or cyclical day-long fasting.

The 5:2 diet, in which you feed regularly for five days and then fast for two days, then alternate-day fasting, in which you fast every other day, are examples of cyclical fasting. Time-restricted fasting simply entails restricting the eating hours to a fixed window during the day, such as eating all of your meals between 10 a.m. – 6 p.m. and fasting for the remaining 16 hours.

Beginning in the early 2000s, animal and laboratory trials of caloric restriction sparked interest in IF as a research subject. Two key biological pathways were discovered to be involved in the development of health benefits from IF in certain animal experiments. One is that IF may trigger ketosis (that you may be acquainted with due to the ketogenic diet), a state in which the body derives energy from stored fats rather than blood sugar (which is usually the body's first go-to source of energy when it requires it). The other mechanism is that cells & tissues may enter a state of rest, regeneration, and rejuvenation, which has been observed in animal studies as well. This could lower the risk of chronic disease and lengthen life expectancy. More of these topics later, but the point is that since research is still in its infancy.

Intermittent fasting is where you just feed during some times of the day. Fasting for some number of hours per day or eating only one meal a couple of times a week will help weight loss. Scientific research also suggests that there are certain health advantages.

Mark Mattson, Ph.D., a neuroscientist at Johns Hopkins University, has practiced intermittent fasting for twenty years. He claims that our bodies have adapted to be capable to go without eating for many hours, days, or even weeks. Hunters and gatherers adapted to live — and grow — for lengthy stretches of time without feeding until humans learned to farm. They needed to: Hunting game and gathering nuts and berries required a lot of time & effort.

It was simpler to keep a healthier weight also 50 years earlier. "There were no phones, only TV programs shut off at 11 p.m.; people avoided consuming before they went to bed," says Christie Williams, M.S.,R.D.N., a dietitian at Johns Hopkins. The portions were much lower. More residents exercised and played outdoors, getting more exercise in general."

Television, the telephone, and other forms of content are now accessible 24 hours a day, seven days a week. We remain up later to watch our favorite movies, play sports, and talk on the internet. We spend the whole day — and much of the night — sitting and snacking."

Type 2 diabetes, Obesity, heart failure, and other diseases may also be exacerbated from eating so much calories and doing so little. Intermittent fasting has been seen in scientific trials to further change these phenomena.

Intermittent fasting is a way of feeding, not a diet. It's a method of planning your meals so can you get the best bang for your buck. Intermittent fasting does not alter your eating habits; however, it alters the timing of your meals.

2.1 Is Intermittent Fasting Worth It?

Most importantly, it's a smart way to get lean while being on a fad diet or severely restricting your calorie intake. In reality, when you first start intermittent fasting, you'll aim to maintain your calorie intake constant. (Most people consume larger meals in a shorter period of time.) Intermittent starvation is often a healthy way to maintain muscle strength when losing weight.

Having said that, the primary motivation for people to pursue intermittent fasting for lose weight. In a second, we'll speak about how intermittent fasting helps you lose weight.

Perhaps notably, since it takes relatively little behaviour adjustment, intermittent fasting is among the best methods we have for losing weight while maintaining a healthy weight. This is a positive thing because it implies intermittent fasting falls under the category of "easy enough to manage, but significant enough to make a difference."

Intermittent fasting (IF) is a form of eating which toggles between fasting & eating times.

It makes no recommendations for items to eat, but rather when you can eat them.

In this way, it's more aptly defined as an eating routine rather than a diet in the traditional sense.

Regular 16-hour fasts and fasting for 24 hrs twice a week are two popular intermittent fasting practices.

Fasting has been practiced by humans since the beginning of time. Supermarkets, refrigerators, and year-round food were not open to ancient hunter-gatherers. They couldn't really find anything to consume.

As a consequence, humans have adapted to be able to survive for long stretches of time without food.

Fasting is, in effect, more normal than consuming 3–4 (or more) meals a day on a regular basis.

Fasting is also practiced in Islam, Christianity, Judaism, and Buddhism for theological or moral purposes.

Intermittent fasting (IF) is a form of eating which alternates between fasting & eating times. It's really common in the health and wellness culture right now.

Chapter 3: Types Of Intermittent Fasting

Diets are becoming more common as a means of losing weight, preventing disease, and increasing longevity. However, depending on your preferences and lifestyle, there are many options.

3.1 Which Kind Of Intermittent Fasting Is Best For You?

"Explain to me what to eat," a registered dietitian always hears. "Tell me what not to eat," they may be hearing now. It's called intermittent fasting (IF) because it's a food strategy that includes interspersing scheduled fasting times with daily meals. This diet, according to proponents, is the secret to long-term weight reduction, improved metabolic fitness, and a long lifespan.

When it comes on weight reduction, there are two theories as to why IF might be successful. The first is that "fasting periods cause a net calorie loss, and as a result, you lose weight," says Rekha Kumar, MD, an endocrinologist, diabetes, and metabolism expert at Weill Cornell Medicine & New York–Presbyterian, New York City. The other definition is more complicated: According to her, this strategy can avoid what is known as the "plateau phenomenon."

You could recall the popular "Biggest Loser" report reported in the journal Obesity in August 2016. After six years, the researchers found that, after the initial remarkable weight loss, the participants had recovered the majority of their weight and that their metabolic activity had slowed, resulting in them burning even fewer calories than would be anticipated.

While the further study on the safety and efficacy of IF is required, one of its touted advantages is that it may avoid metabolic sputtering. "Most individuals who want to lose weight by diet and exercise wind up falling off the wagon and gaining weight." Hormones that stimulate weight gain, such as appetite hormones, are activated, and it's assumed that intermittent fasting (IF) will help avoid this metabolic adaptation," says Dr. Kumar. Normal eating patterns in IF "trick" the body into dropping weight until it reaches a plateau.

No, does it help you lose weight? Proponents of the proposal have agreed in a resounding yes based on anecdotal evidence. "For people who can stick to IF, it works," Kumar says. However, proponents of the method argue that it is about far more than just getting a lean body. Lori Shame, Ph.D., a Dallas diet and weight loss specialist and author of the book Fight with FAT inflammation, tells clients that IF can improve insulin sensitivity (lowering the risk of type 2 diabetes), decrease inflammation, and "boost survival by bettering the health of the mitochondria (cell powerhouses)," according to her.

Obese adults who followed IF for eight weeks lost an average of 10 pounds while also lowering their overall cholesterol, "bad" LDL cholesterol & systolic blood pressure, according to a small study conducted in The US Journal of Clinical Nutrition. The journal Nutrition & Healthy Aging released a report in June 2018 that showed that 3 months of IF didn't impact cholesterol levels, although it did contribute to weight loss and lower systolic blood pressure. In October 2019, the journal Nutrients published a study of 11 IF trials of overweight or obese individuals that lasted at least eight weeks. Nine of those experiments found that an IF regimen was almost as successful at having people shed weight and body fat as conventional dieting instead of cutting calories every day.

However, it's worth noting that researching human lifespan is much more complex than studying weight loss. That's why, like a report released in July 2018 in journal Current Biology, most of the research that says IF encourages a long life has been conducted in animals, including flies. Another study published in the British Medical Journal in December 2019 indicated that the physiological benefit of intermittent fasting is that it puts your body into a condition of ketosis (the keto diet's metabolic state), where fat is burned instead of carbohydrates for energy. According to the researchers, the concept that ketones can activate the body's own repair mechanism, eventually protecting against disease & ageing, goes beyond the weight loss impact.

It's also crucial to keep the hopes in check. Since a lot of testing is focused on animals, it's more challenging to adopt the findings to people who are more free-thinking and have to contend with the consequences of lifestyle problems like job pressures, crazy schedules, emotional eating, and cravings, to list a few — that can make it difficult to stick to a diet. IF might be promising, but it's "actually no more successful than any other diet," according to a 2018 article on the Harvard Health Blog.

3.2 Protocols Of Intermittent Fasting

There are a lot of various ways to do IF, which is fantastic. If this is something you're involved in, you may choose the kind that better suits the needs, increasing your odds of success. Here are seven of them:

5:2 fasting

It is among the most often used IF techniques. In reality, the book The FastDiet popularized it and explained everything you want to know about it. The plan is to diet regularly for five days (without counting calories) and then consume 500-600 calories per day for men and women, respectively, for the remaining two days. The fasting days can be any days you like.

Short fasting periods are thought to keep you compliant; if you get starving on a fast day, think of tomorrow when you will "feast" again. "Some people think, 'I can do something for two days, but cutting down on what I consume for seven days is too much,'" Kumar says. For these individuals, a 5:2 solution could be preferable to calorie restriction during the week.

The Researcher warns against fasting for days where you're performing a lot of intense exercises. If you're practicing for a cycling or running race (or a high-mileage week), see a sports nutritionist see if this style of fasting can fit with your training schedule.

Time-Restricted Fasting

This type of IF allows you to choose an eating window per day, which should leave you with a 14 to 16 hour fast. (Shemek advises women to fast for no longer than 14 hours a day due to hormonal concerns.) "Fasting encourages autophagy, the body's normal 'cellular housekeeping' process that starts when liver glycogen is depleted and clears debris and other items that get in the way of mitochondrial health," Shemek says. According to her, doing so can help maximize fat cell metabolism and optimize insulin function.

Set the eating window, for example, from 9 am-5 pm to make this work. According to Kumar, this works well for anyone with a family who consumes an early dinner anyway. And there's the fact that a lot of the time you're fasting is spent sleeping. (Depending on where you scheduled your window, you still don't have to "skip" any meals.) However, this is contingent on the ability to remain consistent. Regular fasting times might not be for you if your life is constantly shifting or if you need and want the opportunity to go out to brunch on occasion, go on a late date night, and go to happy hour.

Overnight Fasting

This method is the most basic of the bunch, and it entails fasting for 12 hours a day. For instance, choose to avoid eating after dinner at 7 p.m. and start eating at 7 a.m. the next morning with breakfast. At the 12-hour stage, autophagy also occurs, but the cellular benefits are milder, according to Shemek. These are the basic minimum of fasting hour's advice.

This approach has the advantage of being simple to execute. You don't have to miss meals; what you're doing is cutting out a bedtime snack. However, this approach would not fully exploit the benefits of fasting. If you're fasting to lose weight, a narrower fasting window ensures you'll have more time to eat, which may not make you ingest fewer calories.

Eat Stop Eat

This strategy varies from others plans in that it emphasizes versatility. It emphasizes that fasting is simply abstaining from eating for a while. You stick to a resistance conditioning regimen and one or two 24 hr. fasts per week. "When your fast is done, it is suggested to eat responsibly and act as though it never happened. That is what matters in the end.

Eating wisely entails returning to a regular eating routine in which you don't indulge when you've already fasted, but you still don't starve yourself or consume less than you require. Fat reduction is better achieved by combining intermittent fasting with routine weight training, according to Pilon. You will consume a marginally larger number of calories on five to six non-fasting days whether you go on one of two 24-hour fasts throughout the week. This allows it smoother and more fun to finish the week with a calorie shortage without feeling compelled to go on a strict diet.

Whole-Day Fasting

You eat once a day here. According to Shemek, certain individuals choose to eat dinner but then not eat again before the next day's dinner. That means you'll be fasting for 24 hours. This is not the same as the 5:2 form. Fasting times are usually 24 hrs (dinner-dinner or lunch-lunch), while 5:2 needs a 36-hour fast. (For example, you could eat dinner on Sunday, then go on a 500-600 calorie fast on Monday before breaking it with breakfast at Tuesday.)

The benefit is that, if achieved for weight reduction, eating a whole day's worth of calories in single sitting is very difficult (though not impossible). The downside of this strategy is that it's difficult to provide all of the nutrition your body needs with only one meal. Not to mention, sticking to this strategy is difficult. By the time dinner appears, you may be ravenous, leading you to eat less-than-healthy, calorie-dense foods. Consider this: When you're hungry, broccoli isn't the first thing that comes to mind. According to

Shemek, people often consume too much coffee to satisfy their appetite, disrupting their sleep. If you don't eat, you can experience brain fog during the day.

Alternate-Day Fasting

Krista Varady, a nutrition researcher at University of Illinois in Chicago, is popularized this technique. People can fast every other day, where a fast consisting of 25% of their daily caloric needs (approximately 450 calories) and non-fasting days being regular eating days. It is a common weight-loss strategy. In reality, Dr. Varady & colleagues observed that alternate-day fasting was successful in helping elderly persons lose weight in a limited study reported in Nutrition Journal. By week two, the participants' side effects (such as hunger) had subsided, and by week four, they were becoming more satisfied with the diet.

The drawback is that participants claimed they were never really "complete" over the eight weeks of the study, which may render sticking to this plan difficult.

Choose-Your-Day Fasting

It's more of a pick-your-own experience here. According to Shemek, you may undertake time-restricted fasting every other day or maybe once or twice a week (fast for 16 hrs, eat for eight, for example). That means you may have a typical day of eating on Sunday and stop eating by 8 p.m., then start eating again at midday on Monday. It's the equivalent of missing breakfast a couple of times a week.

Something to bear in mind: The data on the impacts of missing breakfast is mixed, according to a study published in the journal Scientific Reviews in Food Science & Nutrition in December 2015. Although some studies demonstrate that consuming it leads to a reduced BMI, there is no consistent evidence in randomized trials that it causes weight reduction. Other studies, such as one published in the American Journal of Cardiology in October 2017, have connected skipping breakfast to lower heart health.

It is more adjustable to your lifestyle and goes with the flow, so you can make it work even if your schedule varies from week to week. However, looser techniques may result in very few improvements.

Fast for straight 12 hours a day

Intermittent fasting may fit different individuals in various ways.

The diet's guidelines are straightforward. Every day, a person must choose and follow a 12-hour fasting pattern.

Fasting for 10–16 hrs, according to some research, causes the body to convert fat storage into energy, releasing ketones into circulation. This should help you lose weight.

For novices, this form of intermittent fasting regimen may be a decent choice. This is because the fasting window is rather limited, most of the fasting happens when sleeping, and the individual may eat the same quantity of calories every day.

The most convenient approach to complete the 12 hrs fast is to include sleep time in the fasting window.

A person might, for example, fast between the hours of 6 p.m. and 6 a.m. They'd have to complete supper before 6 p.m. and wait until 6 a.m. to have breakfast, but they'd be sleeping for most of the time in between.

Fasting for 16 hours

The 16:8 technique, often known as the Leangains diet, involves fasting for 16 hours per day and eating for 8 hours.

Men fast for 16 hrs a day, and women fast about 14 hours on the 16:8 diet. This sort of intermittent fasting may be beneficial for those who have tried the 12-hrs fast and found it ineffective.

People who fast this way generally complete their evening food by 8 p.m., skip breakfast the following day, and don't eat again until midday.

Even though mice ate the same total amount of calories as mice who ate whenever they wanted, research on mice revealed that restricting the feeding window around 8 hours protected them against inflammation, obesity, diabetes, and liver disease.

2 days a week fasting

The 5:2 diet requires people to consume a normal quantity of healthy food for five days and then cut their caloric consumption for the remaining two days.

Men typically ingest 600 calories & women 500 calories during the two fasting days.

Fasting days are usually separated through the week. They may, for example, fast on Mondays and Thursdays and eat regularly for the rest of the week. Between fasting days, there must be at least one non-fasting day.

The 5:2 diet, often known as the Fast diet, has received little investigation. In a research of 107 overweight or obese women, it was shown that calorie restriction twice weekly & continuous calorie restriction both resulted in equivalent weight reduction.

The diet also decreased insulin levels and enhanced insulin sensitivity in the subjects, according to the research.

The results of this fasting technique on 23 overweight women were studied in small-scale research. The ladies dropped 4.8 percent of their overall weight and 8.0 % of their total fat in one menstrual cycle. After 5 days of regular eating, the majority of the women's measures reverted to normal.

Alternate day fasting

The alternate-day fasting strategy, which entails fasting every other day, has various versions.

Some individuals practice alternate-day fasting by avoiding solid meals entirely on fasting days, while others allow up to 500 calories. People often choose to consume as much as they like on feeding days.

According to one research, alternate-day fasting is good for weight reduction and heart health in healthy and overweight individuals, according to Trusted Source. Throughout 12 weeks, the 32 individuals dropped an average of 5.2 kilograms (kg), or slightly over 11 pounds (lb.).

Alternate-day fasting is a more intense type of intermittent fasting that may not be appropriate for novices or people with specific medical issues. In the long run, it may be difficult to continue this form of fasting.

A weekly 24-hour fast

Teas and calorie-free liquids are allowed on a 24-hour diet.

The Eat-Stop-Eat diet entails going without food for 24 hrs at a time for one or two days a week. Many individuals fast from one meal to the next or from one meal to the next.

During the fasting time, people on this diet plan may consume water, tea & other calorie-free beverages.

On non-fasting days, people should resume their usual eating habits. This way of eating lowers a person's overall calorie consumption while leaving the individual's food choices unrestricted.

Fasting for 24 hours may be difficult, leading to weariness, headaches, and irritation. As the body adapts to this new eating pattern, many individuals find that these symptoms become less severe over time.

Before attempting the 24-hour fast, people may benefit from doing a 12-hour or 16-hour fast.

Meal skipping

Beginners may benefit from this radical approach to intermittent fasting. It entails missing meals on occasion.

People may choose which meals to miss based on their hunger levels or time constraints. It is, however, important to consume nutritious meals at each meal.

Individuals who monitor and react to their bodies' hunger cues are more likely to succeed at meal skipping. People who practice intermittent fasting eat when they are starving and skip foods when they are not.

For some individuals, this may feel most natural than the other fasting strategies.

The Warrior Diet

The Warrior Diet is a kind of intermittent fasting that is rather extreme.

Throughout a 20-hrs fasting window, the Warrior Diet entails eating very little, generally only a few portions of raw vegetables and fruit, and then eating one huge meal at night. In most cases, the dining window is just 4 hours long.

This type of intermittent fasting may be appropriate for persons who have previously tried other types of intermittent fasting.

The Warrior Diet advocates argue that humans are naturally nocturnal eaters and that consuming food at night helps the body obtain nutrients according to its circadian cycles.

People should be sure to eat lots of veggies, proteins, and healthy fats throughout the 4-hour meal period. Carbohydrates should also be included.

While it is feasible to consume certain things throughout the fasting period, adhering to the rigorous limits on what and when to eat in long term might be difficult. Furthermore, some individuals find it difficult to consume such a large meal to close tonight.

There's also a chance that folks following this diet won't get adequate nutrients like fibers. It may raise cancer risk and have a negative impact on the immune and digestive systems.

Chapter 4: How Does Intermittent Fasting Work?

Intermittent fasting may be done in various approaches, but they all revolve around selecting regular eating and fasting times. For example, you may try eating just for eight hours a day and fasting for the rest of the day. Alternatively, you might decide to eat just one meal each day, two days per week. There are a variety of intermittent fasting regimens to choose from.

According to Mattson, after a period of time without meals, the body's sugar assets are depleted, and it instigates to burn fat. It is mentioned to as metabolic substituting by scientists.

"Most Americans eat during their waking hours, so intermittent fasting is in contrast to their regular eating pattern," Mattson explains. "If someone eats three meals a day with snacks and doesn't exercise, they're running through those calories but not burning their fat reserves every time they eat."

Intermittent fasting works by extending the time between when your body burns off the calories from your previous meal and starts burning fat.

At its most basic level, intermittent fasting enables the body to utilize its stored energy by burning extra body fat.

It's crucial to remember that this is natural, and people have evolved to be able to fast for shorter periods - hours or days – without experiencing negative health effects.

Food energy has been stored in the form of body fat. Your body will just "consume" its fat for energy if you don't eat.

Life is all about finding the right balance. The yin or the yang, the good & the bad. The same is true when it comes to eating and fasting. After all, fasting is only the opposite of eating. You are fasting if you are not eating.

4.1 The Process Behind IF

When we eat, we consume more food energy than we can utilize right away. Some of this energy will have to be saved for later. Insulin is a hormone that aids in the storage of energy from diet.

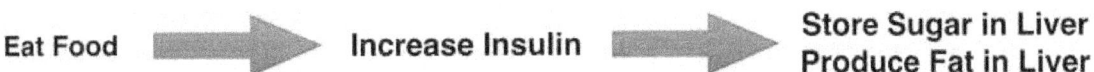

When we eat, our insulin levels increase, assisting us in storing extra energy in two ways. Carbohydrates are digested into glucose (sugar) molecules that may be joined together to produce Glycogen, which is subsequently stored in the muscle or liver.

However, there is a certain amount of storage space for carbs, and once that limit is reached, the liver begins to convert the surplus glucose to fat. De-novo lipogenesis (literally "creating fresh fat") is the name given to this process.

The liver stores some of the newly produced fat, but the majority of it is transferred to other fat deposits throughout the body. Although this is a more difficult procedure, the quantity of fat produced is nearly limitless.

In our bodies, we have two complementary dietary energy storage systems. One is simple to obtain but has limited storage capacity (Glycogen), while the other is relatively difficult to access and has almost infinite storage capacity (glucose) (body fat).

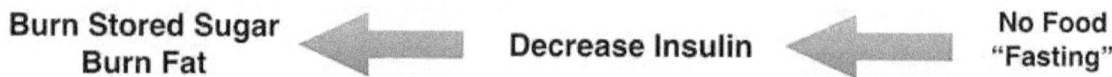

When we don't eat, the process reverses. Insulin levels drop, indicating the body to begin using stored energy because food is no longer available. Because blood glucose levels are dropping, the body must now draw glucose from storage to utilize energy.

The Glycogen is a most readily available energy source. To supply energy to the bodies of other cells, it is broken down into glucose molecules. This may last for 24-36 hours and supply enough energy to meet most of the body's demands. After then, the body's primary source of energy will be the fat breakdown.

So there are only two states in which the body may exist: fed and fasting. We are either accumulating food energy (growing storage) or burning stored energy. It's either this or that. There should be no overall weight change if eating & fasting are equal.

We spend practically all of our lives in the fed state if we start eating as soon as we get out of bed and don't stop unless we go to sleep. We may acquire weight over time because we haven't given our bodies enough time to utilize stored dietary energy.

We may just need to increase the time we spend burning dietary energy to restore equilibrium or reduce weight. Intermittent fasting is what it's called.

Intermittent fasting, in essence, permits the body to utilize its stored energy. What's crucial to remember is that there's nothing wrong with it. That is the way our bodies are made. Dogs, cats, lions & bears all do this. That's what people do.

Your body will continually utilize the incoming food energy if you eat every third hour, as is generally suggested. It may not be necessary to burn much if any, body fat. You may be just accumulating fat.

Your body may be storing it for a period when you won't be able to eat.

If this occurs, you are out of balance. You don't practice intermittent fasting.

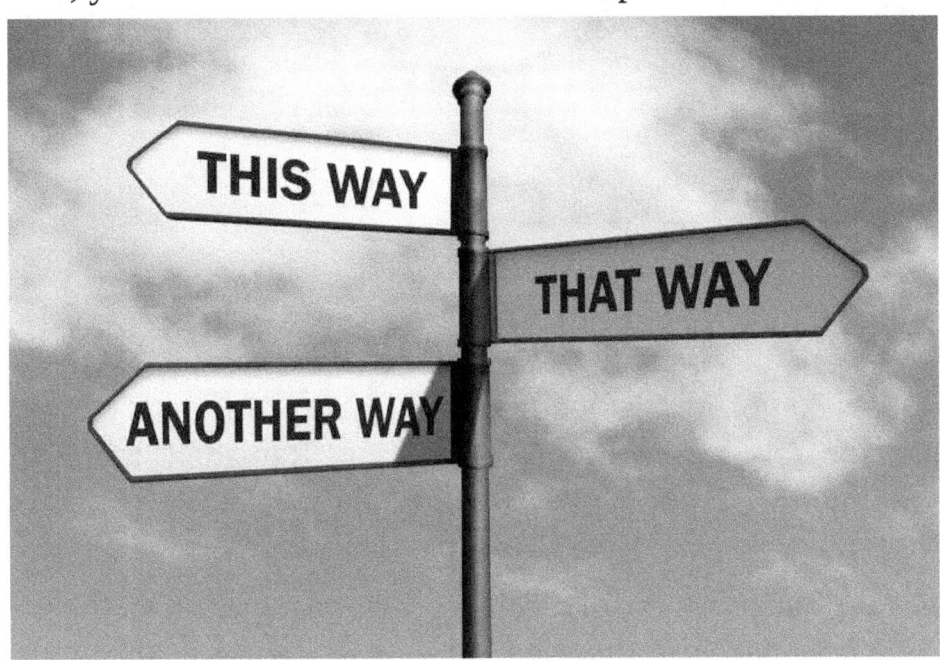

4.2 Short Fasting Regimens – Less Than 24 Hours

Fasting may be done in a variety of ways. But, first and foremost, let's be clear. There is no such thing as a "best" one. For various individuals, all work to varying degrees. There is no right or wrong response, just as some individuals prefer steak over chicken. One individual regimen will be ideal for one individual, while it will be a horrible decision for another.

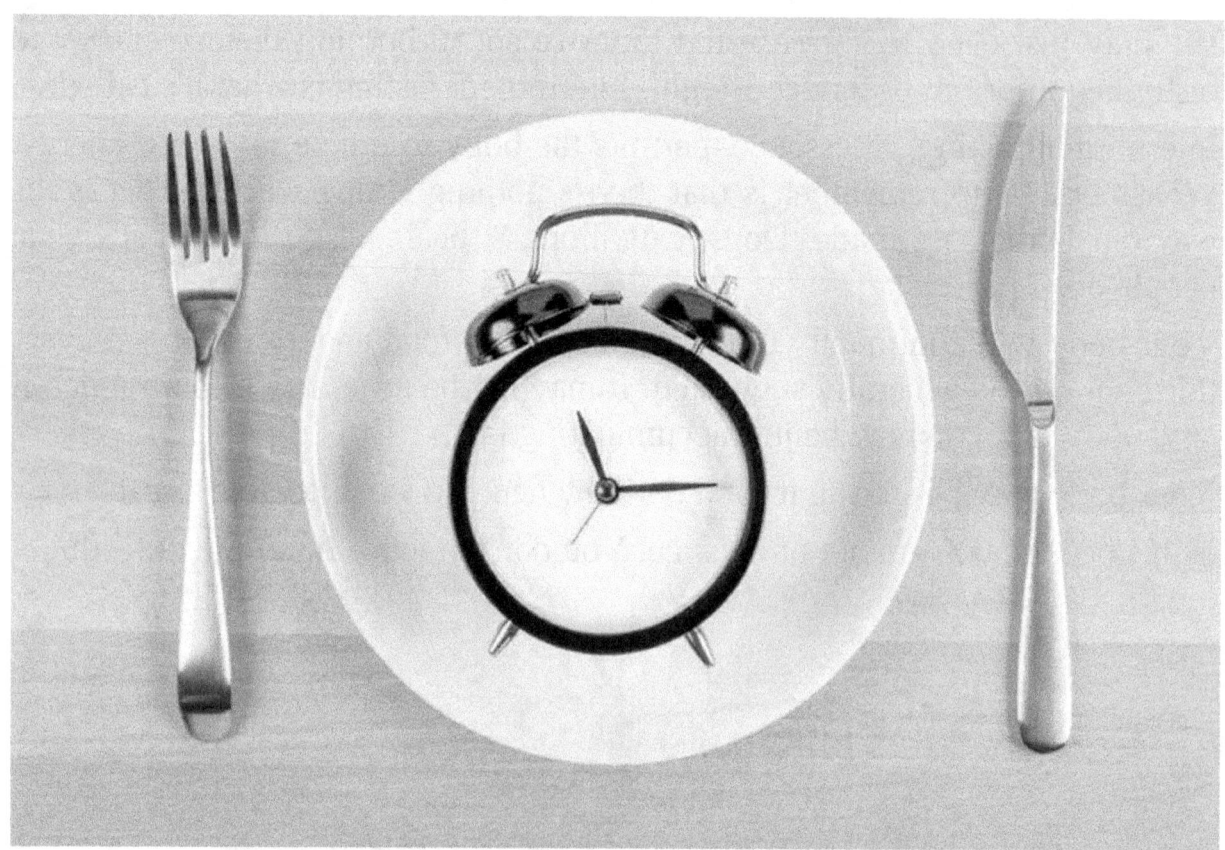

Fasting is the voluntary act of depriving oneself of food for a certain period of time. Water and tea are allowed as non-caloric beverages. An absolute fast is defined as complete abstinence from both food and drink. This is permissible for religious reasons, as during Ramadan there in Muslim religion, although it is not typically advised for health reasons because of dehydration.

Intermittent fasting has a lot of evidence behind it, yet it's still contentious. Medication, particularly for diabetes, poses a risk since dosage must often be adjusted. Talk to your doctor about any medication modifications you've made as well as any lifestyle adjustments you've made.

Those who are skinny or suffer from eating disorders such as anorexia, pregnant or nursing women, and children under 18 should not fast.

4.3 Different Durations

Fasting does not have a set duration. Fasts may last from 12 hours to two months or more (though this is typically not advised!). Once a week, once a month, or once a year, you may fast. Fasting for limited times on a regular basis is known as intermittent fasting. Fasts that are shorter are done more often. Fasts of twenty-four to thirty-six hours are usually done twice or three times a week. Fasting for a lengthy period of time might last anywhere from a week to a month.

All of these fasting regimens have the same goal in mind. It enables the body to reduce insulin levels to dangerously low levels for a longer time than normal. This is exactly what aids in the treatment or prevention of insulin resistance. This is the essential biological concept of homeostasis, as we already said.

Everything in the body prefers to stay inside a small range. As the body strives to resist the change, every extended stimulation causes resistance. In this situation, persistent high insulin levels induce insulin resistance, which causes high insulin levels again — in other words, insulin may produce insulin resistance.

As a result, we may avoid developing insulin resistance and reverse modest degrees of resistance by adding daily or almost daily intervals of low insulin. Longer fasting durations — 24 hours or more – are recommended for more developed resistance.

Although this is rather arbitrary, fasting periods are classified with a breakpoint of 24 hours. Shorter regimens may be used for people who are largely interested in reducing weight without much in form of type-2 diabetes, fatty liver, or other metabolic illnesses, as encountered in the IDM programme.

Longer-duration regimens are required for patients with more serious ailments since they tend to provide quicker benefits. We always work with patients beyond the first' breaking in' stage to determine what they want to do. Longer-duration fasts are preferred by a surprising percentage of patients less often.

4.4 Short Regimens 12-Hour Fasting

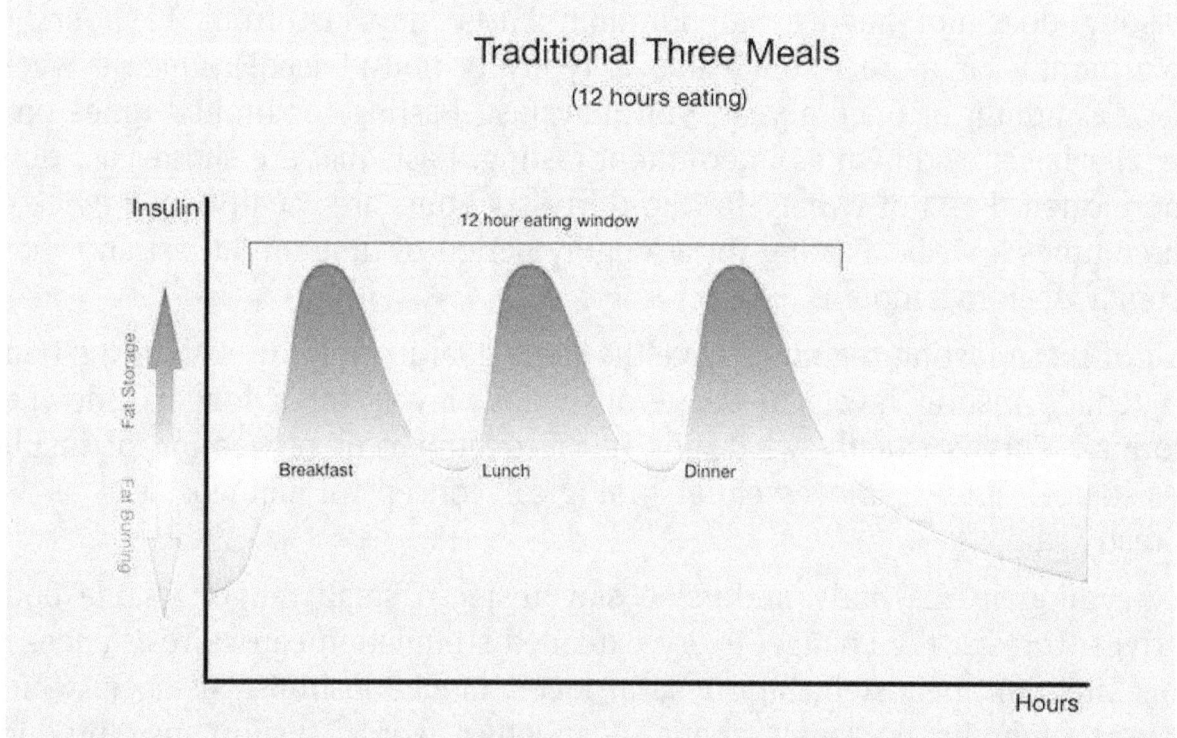

Fasting regimens that involve a shorter duration of fasting but are done every day are possible. It used to be considered normal to fast for 12 hours every day. That is, you could eat three meals a day from 7 a.m. to 7 p.m. and then fast from 7 p.m. to 7 a.m.

You'd eat a small breakfast to 'break your fast' at that point. In the 1950s & 1960s, this was very common. Back then, there wasn't a lot of obesity. However, there have been two significant developments since then. The first was switching to a lower-fat, higher-carbohydrate diet. Insulin levels and hunger levels both increased as a result of this. The second factor was an increase in meal frequency, which tended to shorten fasting times, as we discussed in a previous piece.

This 12-hour daily fasting proved probably excellent enough for most individuals to prevent obesity provided they could consume unprocessed meals, avoid excessive added sugars, plus did not have severe insulin resistance, to begin with. It is, however, insufficient to repair decades of insulin resistance.

4.5 16-Hour Fasting

Intermittent fasting, often known as 16:8, is a kind of time-restricted fasting. It entails eating for 8 hours and then fasting for the remaining 16 hrs of the day.

Some individuals feel that this practice helps the body's circadian rhythm or internal clock perform better.

The 16:8 diet requires most individuals to fast at night and for a portion of the morning & evening. They eat the majority of their calories in the mid of the day.

During the 8-hour interval, there are no limits on the types or quantities of food that may be consumed. The strategy is reasonably simple to follow because of this flexibility.

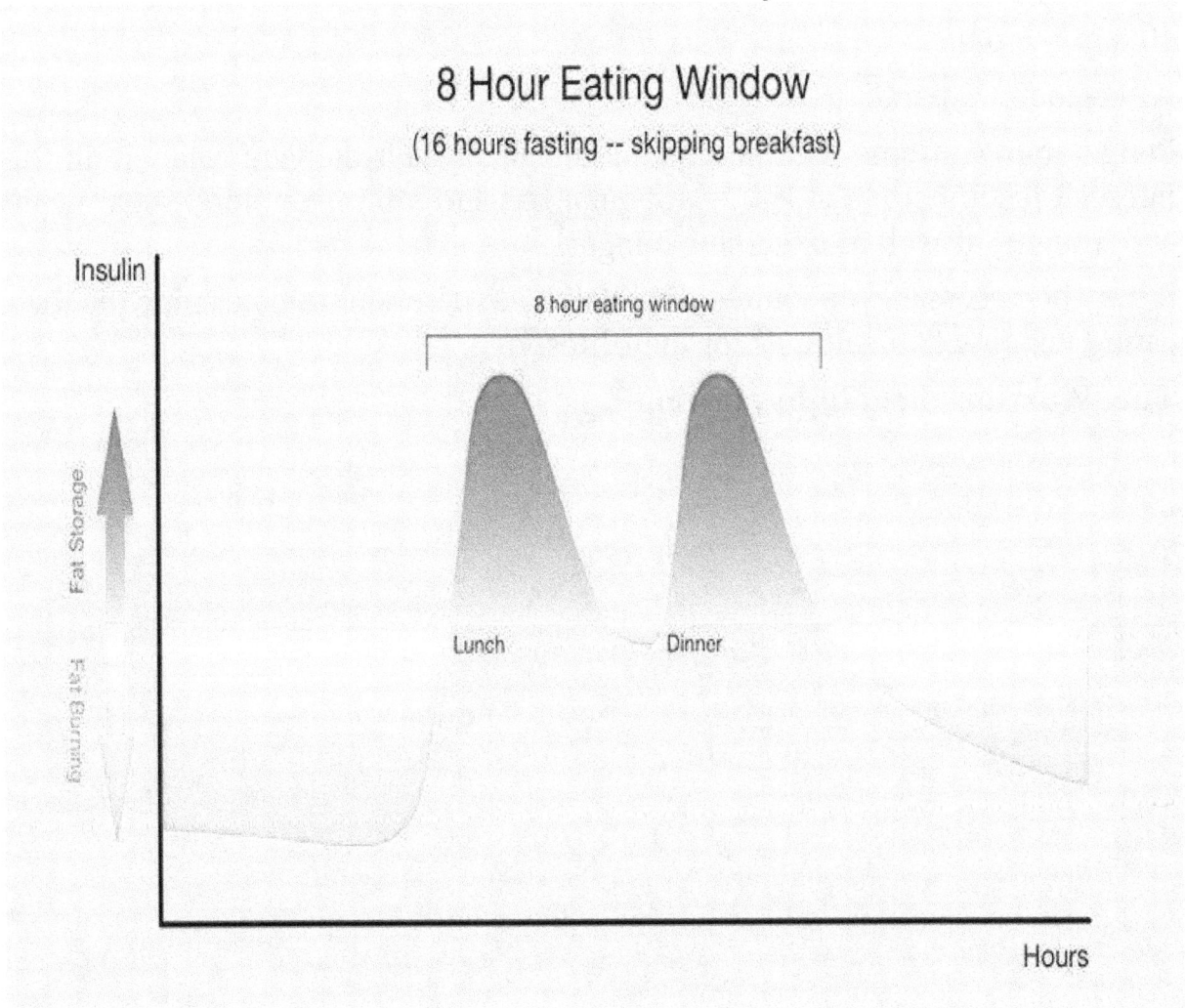

This plan calls for a 16-hour fast followed by an 8-hour 'eating window'

every day. This would entail eating from 11 a.m. to 7 p.m. and fasting from 7 p.m. to 11 a.m. This usually entails missing breakfast every day. Some individuals consume two meals over eight hours, while others eat three.

The best approach to stick to the 16:8 diet is to pick a 16-hour fasting period that includes sleep time.

Some experts recommend completing your meal in the early evening since your metabolism slows down after that. This is not, however, practicable for everyone.

Some individuals may not be able to eat until 7 p.m. and later in the evening. Even so, it's preferable to fast for 2–3 hours before going to bed.

People may eat during one of the eight-hour eating periods listed below:

9 a.m. - 5 p.m.

10 a.m. - 6 p.m.

After-noon - 8 p.m.

People may consume their snacks and meals at their convenience within this interval. It's important to eat on a regular basis to minimize blood sugar peaks and troughs, as well as excessive hunger.

It may be necessary for some individuals to experiment to determine the ideal eating window & mealtimes for their lifestyle.

The 'Warrior' diet (20-hrs fasting)

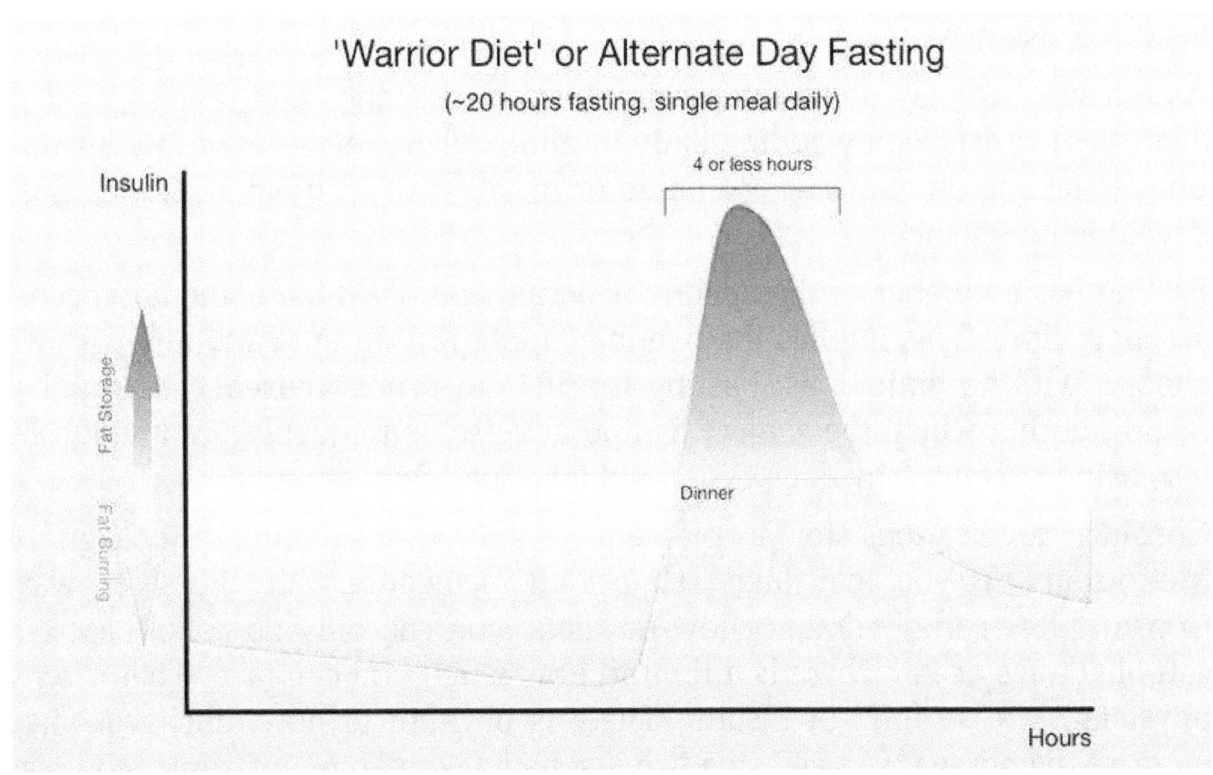

Intermittent fasting was popularized by this diet, which was one of the earliest to do so. This diet emphasized that mealtime was nearly as important as meal content. To put it another way, 'when you eat, what you eat becomes essential.'

The diet's core consists of eating meals in the evening within a 4-hour window, drawing inspiration from historic warrior cultures such as the Spartans and Romans. The fasting period lasted 20 hours and included most of the day. A Natural, unadulterated diet and high-intensity exercises were also emphasized.

4.6 What's The Point Of Incorporating Daily Fasting?

All of these fasting regimens have the same goal in mind. It enables the body to reduce insulin levels to dangerously low levels for a longer time than normal. This is exactly what aids in the treatment or prevention of insulin resistance. This is the essential biological concept of homeostasis, as we already said.

Everything in the body prefers to stay inside a small range. As the body strives to resist the change, every extended stimulation causes resistance. In this situation, persistent high insulin levels induce insulin resistance, which causes high insulin levels again — in other words, insulin may produce insulin resistance.

As a result, we may avoid developing insulin resistance and reverse modest degrees of resistance by adding daily or almost daily intervals of low insulin. Longer fasting durations — 24 hours or more – are recommended for more developed resistance.

Fasting has a number of therapeutic benefits, one of which is the absence of an upper limit. This implies that we may apply fasting in nearly any way we choose, with no limitations. Fasting for 382 days (not advised!) set a global record, during which the subject had no adverse consequences (Although he was being examined by doctors and did take specific vitamins).

Consider medications for a moment. There is a maximum dosage of Metformin that you may take. Almost all medications are the same way. Consider low-carbohydrate or low-fat diets: you can only go as low as zero carbohydrates or fat. There is a limit to how much you can take. That is why physicians are so fond of insulin. There is no limit to how much you may increase the dosage. (As an aside, we just had a woman in our clinic who was on 400 units of insulin each day.) Her endocrinologist was relieved that her blood sugar levels were now under control.)

Fasting, too, has no upper limit, allowing for more therapeutic flexibility. To put it another way, you may maintain fasting until you get the desired result. The dosage may be increased indefinitely. Will you lose weight if you don't eat? Yes, of course. As a result, effectiveness is essentially a non-issue. It's only a matter of being safe and following the rules. We may simply raise the dosage in more difficult or dangerous instances.

Longer fasting regimens – 24 hrs or maybe more

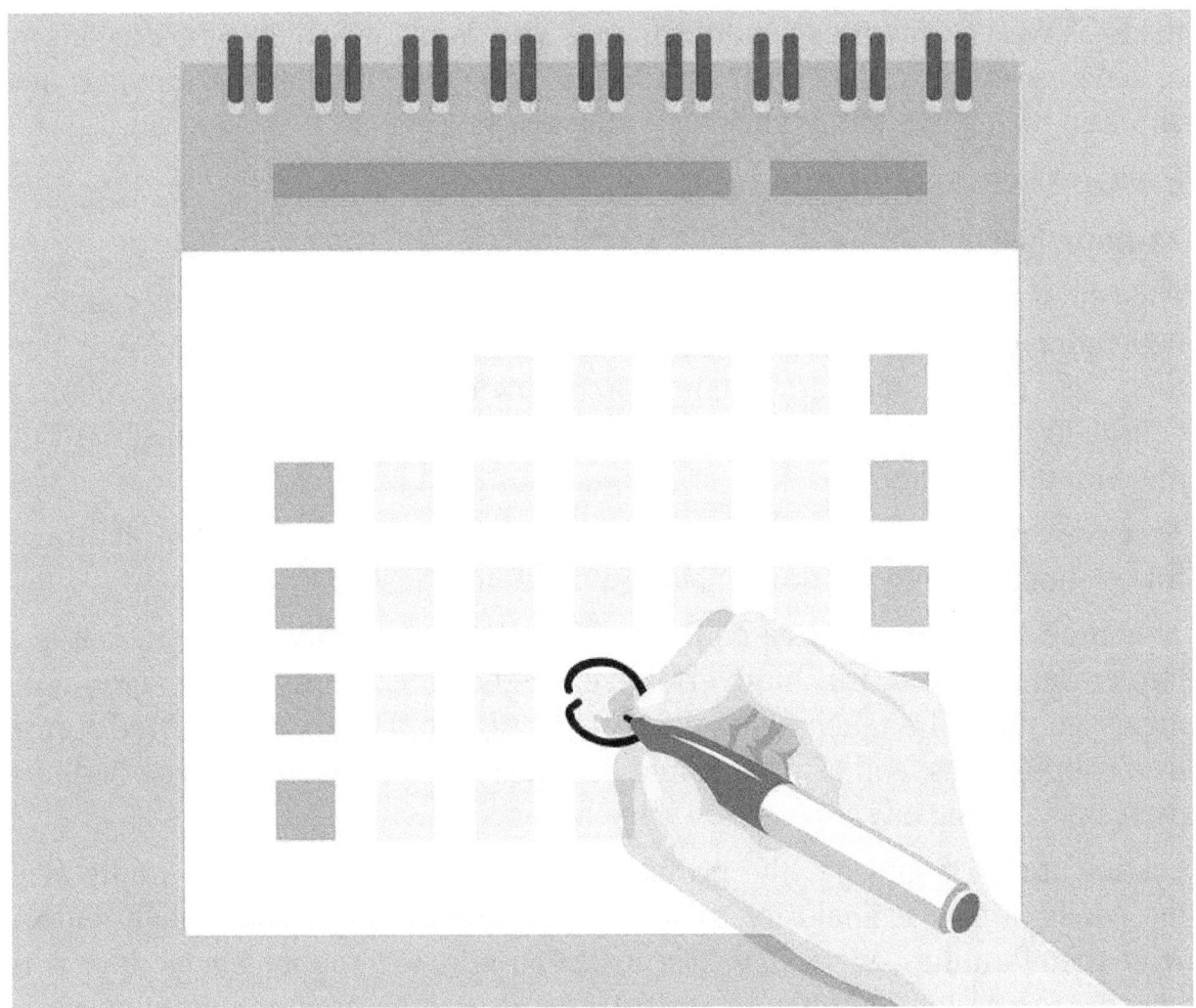

It is divided at 24 hours randomly, though there is no physiological rationale for this other than categorization considerations. There is no such thing as a magical dividing line.

Fasting regimens with durations of fewer than 24 hours were discussed. Longer regimens are usually followed less regularly. Personal choice is the most important factor in determining which fasting regimen is best for you. Longer fasts are easy for some individuals and difficult for others.

The majority of individuals experience an increase in hunger on day two. Hunger peaks at that moment and then gradually fades. If you're planning on doing a longer fast, you'll need to know this (3-7 days). It's simpler to keep going when you know that hunger will subside over time.

Intermittent fasting has a lot of evidence behind it, yet it's still contentious. Medication, particularly for diabetes, poses a risk since dosage must often be adjusted. Talk to your doctor about any medication modifications you've made as well as any lifestyle adjustments you've made. Those who are skinny or have eating disorders such as anorexia, pregnant mothers or nursing, and children under 18 should not fast.

Fasting sessions of one long day

24-hour fasts

A 24-hour fast might go from dinner to dinner or from breakfast to breakfast, depending on your preference. For example, you may eat dinner at 7 p.m. and then fast until dinner at 7 p.m. the following day. You do not spend a complete day without eating on this regimen since you still consume one meal on the 'fasting' day.

This is extremely similar to the 'Warrior' fasting approach. However, it allows for a 4-hour feeding window, making it a 20-hour fast.

This time of fasting offers a number of significant benefits. First, since it is a longer-duration fast, it is more effective. Medication that has to be taken with meals may still be taken since you eat every day. For example, Metformin, iron supplements, and aspirin should be taken with meals and maybe had one meal on a fasting day.

Fasting for 24 hours has the primary benefit of being simple to implement into daily life. The majority of individuals, for example, will have supper with their families every day. Because you still eat supper every day, it is feasible to fast for 24 hours on a regular basis without anybody noticing since it only entails missing lunch and breakfast on that particular day.

This is especially simple throughout the daytime. You just have a cup of coffee in the morning and skip breakfast. You work through lunch and, once again, get home in time for supper. This saves time as well as money. Breakfast does not need any cleaning or preparation. You spare an hour at lunchtime to work and then return home for supper without anybody noticing you'd been fasting for 24 hours.

The reduction of lean body mass, and muscle, is one of the most common concerns associated with fasting. Many research has been conducted on this topic, and these fears are mostly unfounded, particularly among overweight or obese people. According to one research, fasting every other day for 22 days did not reduce lean body mass, even while body weight decreased significantly.

OMAD, or One Meal A Day, is another term for a similar fast.

The 5:2 diet

While pioneers like Martin Berkhan & Brad Pilon had sparked some interest on the fringes, fasting had not yet reached the mainstream. With the BBC broadcast and the book that followed, there were many buzzes, particularly in the UK.

The basic diet did not include a full 24-hour fast. The 5:2 diet consists of 5 days of regular eating followed by 2 days of fasting. You might consume total 500 calories on the other two days. Those 500 calories might be consumed in one sitting. If this were had as dinner, it would be equivalent to a 24-hour fast. You may, however, divide those 500 calories throughout many meals. These two procedures are quite similar, and the physiological differences are expected to be minor.

4.7 Alternate Daily Fasting (ADF)

This is the dietary regimen with the greatest scientific support. Dr. Krista Varady, an associate professor of nutrition at the University of Illinois – Chicago, was responsible for most of it.

Even though it seems that you only eat the second day, this is not the truth. On fasting days, you may consume up to 500 calories, exactly as on the 5:2 diet. On the other hand, fasting days are conducted on alternate days instead of twice a week, making it a more severe routine.

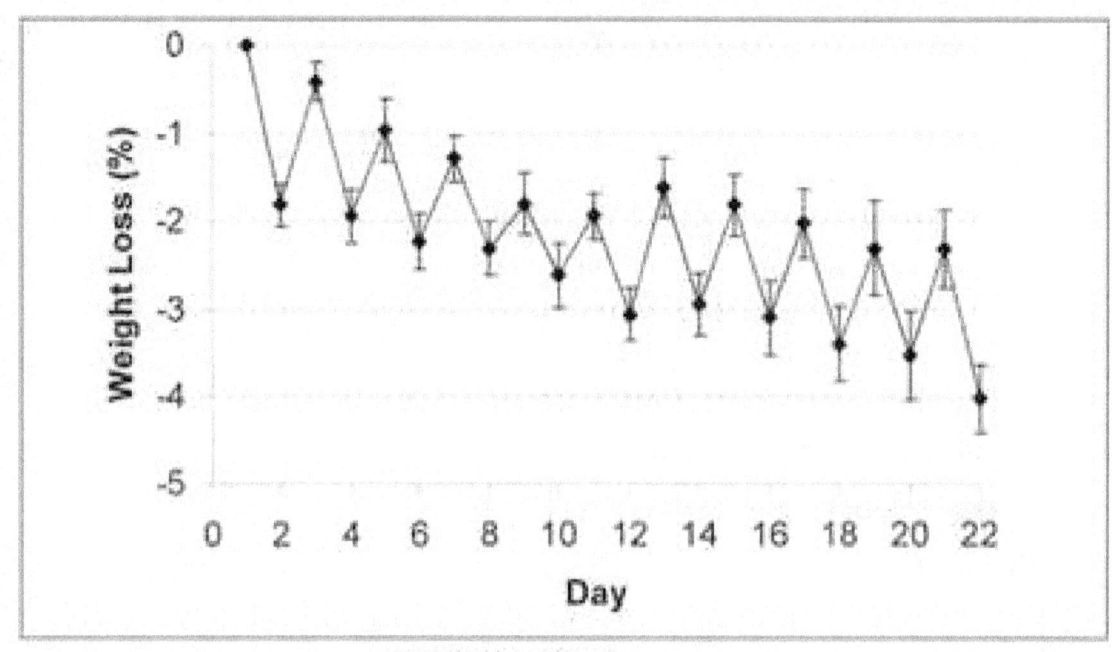

Heilbronn LK et al
Am J Clin Nutr 2005;81:69-73.

4.8 Complications Risk Of Fasts >24 Hours

Fasting for extended periods of time provides additional advantages, but it also increases the risk of problems.

Another important factor to remember is that a doctor must closely manage medicine. The biggest issue is diabetes drugs since if you consume the same dosage and don't eat, you'll get hypoglycemia, which is hazardous.

Low blood sugar is not a problem in and of itself since it is usually the objective of fasting. We wish the sugar levels to drop. It does, however, imply that you got overmedicated on that particular day. To alter prescriptions and check glucose, you'll need to work closely with your doctor. Additionally, several drugs may induce stomach distress if taken on an empty stomach. ASA, NSAIDs, iron supplements & Metformin, are the most often prescribed medications.

To prevent hypoglycemia, diabetes medications and insulin must be lowered on fasting days. Your doctor should determine how much you should lower it.

It is not advised for anybody on medication to attempt lengthier fasts without first seeing their doctor.

36-hour fasts

A 36-hour fast is equivalent to a one-day fast. For example, suppose you complete dinner at 7 p.m. on day 1, skip all meals on day 2, and don't eat again till breakfast at 7 a.m. on day 3. So you've fasted for a total of 36 hours.

For type 2 diabetes, we often suggest 36-hour fasts 2-3 times a week at our clinic. This prolonged fasting time, in my experience, delivers faster benefits while maintaining high compliance. Because type 2 diabetics have increased insulin resistance, a long fasting period is more helpful than a series of shorter fasts, but we've seen excellent success with both.

42-hour and beyond fasts

We often urge our customers to create a habit of preceding breakfast and breaking their fast around midday. This makes it simple to adhere to a 16:8 fasting schedule on a regular basis. Most individuals begin to feel pretty normal after a few days of just beginning their day with the glass of water and customary cup of coffee.

When you combine a 36-hour fast to it, you get a 42-hr fasting period. On day 1, for example, you would have dinner at 6 p.m. On day 2, you miss all meals and have your customary "breakfast" meal at midnight. This adds up to 42 hours.

When it comes to longer-term fasts, we frequently aim to avoid calorie restriction throughout the feeding time. We often hear that when individuals get used to fasting, their hunger begins to wane. Not at all. Down is the word. On their eating day, they should eat till they are satisfied.

This decrease in appetite has a very excellent explanation. Insulin levels begin to fall as you begin to break your insulin resistance cycle. Hunger is repressed as a result, and total energy expenditure is maintained. As a result, appetite decreases while TEE remains constant or increases. Remember that persistent daily calorie restriction has the opposite effect. TEE decreases when appetite rises, resulting in subpar performance.

Fasts may be made considerably longer. Although the world record for fasting is 382 days (not advised!), many individuals can fast for 7-14 days without issue. Indeed, Beyonce's Master Cleanse is a 7-day fast with the addition of maple syrup, lemonade and cayenne pepper combination.

There are some potential advantages to promoting autophagy, a cellular cleansing process that frequently requires fasting for 48 hours or longer. To enter ketosis, you may need to fast for more than 36 hours. Theoretically, there are several advantages, including hunger control and improved mental clarity. Some recommend a seven-day fast for cancer prevention. However, many of these advantages are hypothetical and untested. Nonetheless, many people have found a 7-day fast to be considerably easier than they had expected.

Chapter 5: Intermittent Fasting For Women After 50

When it comes to losing weight, women over 50 often have a difficult time. A variety of factors may cause this. The most common cause is a slowed metabolism. The quicker your metabolism is, the more muscle mass you have. However, as we age, we lost lean muscle mass and became less active than we once were. What's the result? Stubborn body fat that refuses to go away.

Women over 50 may benefit from intermittent fasting to lose weight and reduce their risk of acquiring age-related disorders.

Lower metabolism, achy joints, diminished muscle mass, and even sleep troubles make it more difficult to lose weight beyond 50. Simultaneously, decreasing fat, particularly harmful belly fat, may significantly lower your chance of major health problems, including diabetes, heart attacks & cancer.

Of course, as you become older, your chances of contracting a variety of diseases rise. When it comes to weight reduction and reducing the risk of acquiring age-related disorders, intermittent fasting for older women may be a veritable fountain of youth in certain circumstances.

Intermittent fasting has grown in popularity in recent years due to its many health advantages and the fact that it does not limit your meal choices. According to research, fasting has been shown to boost metabolism, mental health, and perhaps prevent various cancers. It may also protect women over 50 against certain muscle, neural, and joint diseases.

5.1 Key Benefits Of Intermittent Fasting For Over 50 Women

The benefits of IF go beyond weight reduction. Fasting has been performed in certain societies since ancient times, and it is currently done regularly in others.

Health advantages are a nice side effect of IF, but many of them are beneficial to women's health in particular.

- **Musculoskeletal health:** Arthritis, Osteoporosis, and lower back discomfort are all examples of this. Fasting has been found to increase thyroid hormone output. It may help avoid bone fractures by promoting bone health.

- **Metabolic health:** In their 50s, some women experience menopause. Changes in your body during menopause might lead to an increase in belly fat, insulin, & glucose levels. Fasting may help you lose weight and increase insulin sensitivity by lowering blood pressure, cholesterol, & belly fat. Fasting may also help you maintain a healthy metabolism as you become older.
- **Mental health:** Fasting has been proved to be beneficial to one's mental health. It may help with anxiety, despair, and the emotional ups and downs that come with menopause. Fasting has also been shown to boost self-esteem and lower stress levels.

IF has also been shown to have the following advantages:

- Tissue health
- Improved memory
- Heart health
- Physical performance

5.2 Women Over 50 May Extend Beyond Calorie Restriction

While some nutritionists believe that IF works because it encourages individuals to eat less, others disagree, they think that with the same quantity of calories & other nutrients, intermittent fasting produces greater benefits than traditional meal patterns. Studies have also shown that fasting for many hours a day accomplishes more than simply calorie restriction.

These are among the metabolic alterations that IF generates, which may help explain the synergistic effects:

- **Insulin:** Lower insulin levels throughout the fasting phase will aid fat burning.
- **HGH:** HGH levels increase when insulin levels fall, promoting fat burning and muscle building.
- **Noradrenaline:** The neurological system will transmit this molecule to cells in reaction to an empty stomach, informing them that they must release fat for fuel.

5.3 Typical Results Of Intermittent Fasting

Dr. Becky, a chiropractor, and over-50 fitness specialist, says it's difficult to uncover any drawbacks to IF in the medical literature. She emphasized that your blood sugar & insulin levels would drop to dangerously low levels during the fasting period. Your body will depend on stored fat for energy if insulin's hormonal fat-storing signal is not present.

The National Library of Medicine has also provided a summary of women's health-related intermittent fast outcomes. Studies on using fasting as a technique to lower the risk of cancer, diabetes, and other metabolic disorders, as well as heart disease, are among the report's highlights.

5.4 Intermittent Fasting As Best Fat-Loss Tool

In any event, IF seems to function mostly because it is quite simple to follow. By restricting meal windows, they claim, helps individuals organically control calories and make healthier food choices. According to several research, IF tends to boost fat loss while conserving lean muscle mass, making it a better option than just lowering calories, carbohydrates, or fat.

Of course, the majority of individuals combine IF with some other weight-loss strategy. To reduce weight, you can decide to consume 1,200 calories each day. It may be better to spread out 1,200 kcal across two meals and two snacks rather than three meals and three snacks. If you've had trouble losing weight because your diet didn't work or was too difficult to keep to, you may want to try intermittent fasting.

Dr. Kathryn Waldrep suggests eating within an 8 hrs window and picking that period based on your body's circadian cycles in Prime Women's freshly released PLATE, an intermittent fasting program. Eat between 9 a.m. to 5 p.m. if you're an early riser. Night owls would consume their first meal about midday and their final meal at 8:00 p.m. There seems to be convincing evidence on the efficacy of this method to eating for weight control as more study on IF and circadian rhythms is conducted.

Chapter 6: Considering Factors Before Trying IF

Many advocates believe that intermittent fasting is more than simply a fleeting trend. The history of humanity has shown that empires often last extended periods. There are several religions, including many of the world's largest religious groups, which practice periods of fasting, such as during Lent. Although our predecessors were forced to endure intermittent fasting because of how they obtained food, this kind of food availability was normal for them because of their hunting-gathering lifestyle.

Several years ago, the attention of the public was turned to the subject of fasting once again. The excitement in fasting has increased significantly over the years since it is yet another diet claimed to assist individuals in shed excess pounds with the hopes of improving their health and look. Like all diets, there are staunch proponents and vocal critics, with some individuals finding it difficult to sustain for an extended period.

It's important to distinguish intermittent fasting from other trendy diet fads. While many faiths and cultures have benefitted from a healthy meditation practice throughout history, meditation itself is not always practiced healthily, with no rules or guidelines. This is interesting, to say the least since the public's interest in it has been heightened over the last several years.

Similar to previous trends like intermittent fasting, there are risks, and intermittent fasting should not be used as a strategy for weight loss for everyone. Widespread changes in eating habits, such lengthy periods of fasting, during pregnancy, and those who are recovering from eating disorders and diabetes are potentially dangerous. Pregnant women and patients with diabetes should often eat modest portions of food, particularly when they are under a lot of stress. It may be detrimental to their health if they go without food for 16 hours. It is usually a good idea to see a dietician before making any changes to your diet.

Instead of focusing on what to eat, this fasting pattern doesn't concern itself with when to eat. A consistent eating pattern consists of intermittent fasting, with eating patterns also varying depending on how long the fast lasts. Intermittent fasting is giving up eating for varying lengths of time on certain days of the week. In the last decade, the most popular diet trends have been those that claim to lead to improved health, more concentration, more energy, and the reduction of some inches. It is necessary to find out what you're getting yourself into before deciding to adopt an intermittent fasting meal plan.

Some people claim that intermittent fasting (also called "time-restricted feeding" or "intermittent fasting") may have some health advantages, but to plunge directly into an intermittent fast is not advised, according to Dr. Kahan. Regardless of the reason you're contemplating fasting, it's always a good idea to speak with your doctor about it before trying it out, he adds. A short period of time without food allows the body to detoxify and improve its overall functioning.

Fasting promotes fat burning

Intermittent fasting offers the hope & promise of becoming fitter and healthier, claims Mattson. Your body utilizes up the glucose stored in your liver as a source of energy while fasting. "Next, you use your stored fat as your primary source of energy." Ketosis is a condition characterized by increased ketone levels. It often results in weight loss. It's believed that the three-meals-a-day eating schedule followed by Americans plus their snacks don't give the body the time to use the liver's energy reserves and make the transition to fat-burning, as he suggests.

Fasting provides mental clarity

According to Mattson, a study demonstrates that intermittent fasting has been shown to enhance working memory in animals and verbal memory in adults. He notes a study involving 220 healthy, non-obese people who were instructed to follow the calorie-restricted diet for two years. Results indicated evidence of better memory in the battery of cognitive tests. Although the process by which fasting enhances memory is not completely known, further study is underway, according to him.

Fasting promotes weight reduction.

But this seems to be just temporary, according to Dr. Kahan. Going back to your old eating habits after a period of fasting is likely to result in regaining all or a portion of weight that you lost. In the research mentioned above, it was shown that fasting is capable of causing short-term weight reduction and reducing cholesterol levels in the blood for just a short period of time. The panel recommended that there is not enough data to establish if it is useful for the long run.

Fasting may provide health advantages

Much of the study on fasting has been performed with animals, and it isn't easy to apply this information to humans. There is an increasing body of scientific literature on the relationship between fasting and human health. This literature concludes that some kinds of fasting may improve your cholesterol, blood sugar, blood pressure, or glucose levels and help control other conditions such as insulin sensitivity. While the advantages of intermittent fasting could be different for women, you should be aware of these differences.

Routine fasters may have a long life

As the results of two recent research presented at the 2019 conference of the US Heart Association are showing. A five-year-long routine fast was used in one cardiac patient research, including "routine fasters" (patients who had been fasting consistently for at least five years). A 45% lower chance of dying was seen among the fasters, who were assigned a daily exercise plan, during the subsequent 12 years compared to the non-fasters. The research was placed in Utah and other Rocky Mountain states & included Mormons, church members of Jesus-Christ of Latter-day Saints (also referred to as Mormons), who fast on Sundays and eat food provided by the church other five days of the month.

The results of a second similar trial revealed regular fasting decreased the risk of heart failure by 71 percent in those who did not already have heart failure. The research was observational, so it does not show cause and effect, but the findings may or may not result from a healthy lifestyle, and the timing of the findings might indicate whether fasting is an indication of such a lifestyle or is responsible for other good changes.

Side effects may occur with fasting.

Regardless of the form of fasting you choose, you may experience headaches, fainting, weakness, & dehydration. Risks might vary depending on the fast. Dr. Kahan mentions that certain juice fasts may put people at risk for kidney stones, for example.

Your stomach will be growling...for the first time

Since the 1970s, Mattson has had brief bursts of improvement. In addition to eating less calories, meal skipping is also known as fasting. Starting by missing breakfast causes you to feel hungry in the morning, but you will no longer be hungry in the morning after a few weeks.

What you consume before and then after a fast will impact your weight loss goals.

The American College of Physicians, which consists of over 27,000 physicians, recommend eating healthful meals before a fast, like fruits, vegetables, & lean protein, while avoiding items that are heavy in salt, which may promote bloating. Once you have finished your fast, you should begin to gradually add meals to help you avoid an overeating incident. To know more about what you're permitted to drink throughout the fast, read more here.

Fasting may have a positive effect on the structure of the body.

People who have issues with their weight could benefit from a structured diet where foods are structured and delivered for a particular period of time. "If you have a strict set of restrictions, such as 'people only allowed to eat between the hours of 11 a.m. and 6 p.m.,' that might be a beneficial structure," Dr. Kahan explains. You will profit if you can accomplish things like that fairly, and when it comes to food, you make healthy selections. When individuals start to believe that fasting is wonderful & that they can eat anything they want during such periods because their body is like a fat-burning engine, the complications emerge.

Not everyone is suited to fasting.

The list of people as they should not fast includes under 25, pregnant women or breastfeeding, individuals with diabetes and taking medication to control blood sugar, individuals with seizure disorders, and those who work in a job requiring them to operate heavy machinery. Dr. Kahan cautions that you should avoid intermittent fasting, regardless of whether you have an eating order. When you have an eating problem such as binge-eating disorder, any restricted eating tends to lead to increased bingeing, he explains.

"Are you enjoying this book? If so, I'd be really happy if you could leave a short review on Amazon, it means a lot for me! Thank You"

DOWNLOAD NOW A FREE COPY OF

"7 Days Meal Plan For Intermittent Fasting"

[Click Here](#)

Chapter 7: What Intermittent Fasting Does and Doesn't Do?

Intermittent fasting is not a new concept, despite the word being a recent creation. What's new is that clinical studies regarding IF's health and lifespan advantages are now catching up.

If you're trying to lose weight, the diet that emphasizes when you eat rather than what you eat may be an excellent strategy to reduce weight while also improving your cardiovascular health.

Anyone who has tried a variety of weight-loss regimens is likely aware with their drawbacks. Low-calorie diets can make you exhausted, hungry, and irritable. Cravings and constipation are common side effects of low-carb or "keto" diets. Low-fat diets are extremely difficult to stick to, and they do not seem to protect against cardiovascular disease, contrary to common perception.

Intermittent fasting, another popular diet fad, takes a different method. This diet restricts when you eat rather than what you consume. According to Dr. Eric Rimm, professor of medicine and nutrition at Harvard National Institute Of Public Health, some individuals may find the shift simpler to manage.

According to short-term research, intermittent fasting diets seem to be as effective as or better than conventional diets. Intermittent fasting increases weight reduction and may lower risk factors connected to heart diseases, such as diabetes, high blood pressure, abnormal blood lipid levels, and inflammation, according to a review paper published in the journal Nutrients in 2019.

"However, we don't have much information regarding how this diet works over time," Dr. Rimm adds, adding that just two long-term trials of intermittent fasting, every lasting a year, exist. There are also no huge groups of individuals who have been eating this way for a long time. The Mediterranean diet & a vegetarian diet, on the other hand, have been related to a healthy heart and body size.

Is there an evolutionary benefit here?

Those who are overweight or obese, however, may choose to attempt intermittent fasting. According to Dr. Rimm, this diet has certain distinctive elements that may explain its effectiveness, in addition to its obvious heart-related advantages. First and foremost, the approach makes evolutionary sense. Food resources fluctuated in abundance and scarcity as early people developed. We developed in lockstep with the environmental day-night cycle as well. As a result, our metabolism evolved to work best when we were hungry and eating throughout the day, and resting at night. Many studies have connected late-night snacking to weight gain & diabetes, and one study even revealed that men who snacked late at night had a greater risk of heart attack than those who didn't.

Second, intermittent fasting emphasizes some of the benefits of other diet plans while avoiding the drawbacks. "People who practice whole-day or alternate-day fasting rapidly learn how many calories particular meals contain. It enables individuals to choose meals that are both full and low in calories, "Dr. Rimm believes. The diet is simpler to sustain since they aren't constantly monitoring calories and feeling starved every day.

7.1 Burning Stored Fat

Fasting on a regular basis promotes the same fat-burning process as a keto diet or low-carbohydrate. The metabolic process that occurs when your body loses glucose (its primary energy source) and begins to burn stored fat is known as ketosis. After only 12 hrs of not eating, your body may enter ketosis, which many individuals do overnight before "breakfast" with the morning meal. (Obviously, a late-night snack thwarts this plan.) Because you avoid carbs, which provide glucose, a keto diet maintains people in ketosis for much longer. Fat, on the other hand, becomes the primary fuel source.

However, other nutritionists are concerned that keto diets, which often contain many meat and eggs, might be harmful to the heart. Intermittent fasting is likely to be a healthier alternative, particularly if you consume a well-balanced diet that includes nuts, legumes, fruits, whole grains, and vegetables, all of which are high in nutrients that have been linked to a reduced risk of heart disease.

Intermittent fasting regimens, on the other hand, don't usually stipulate what items you should consume. "That makes me a bit uneasy as a nutritional epidemiologist," Dr. Rimm confesses. He thinks it's not good to eat burgers & French fries 5 days a week and a single breakfast sandwich on a low-calorie day. However, like with any diet, it's best to ease into the adjustments. Start with a 5:2 diet or a time-restricted eating plan. He says that after you start reducing weight, you may gradually incorporate more nutritious meals.

However, don't anticipate immediate results. People who use intermittent fasting lose weight slowly, approximately half a pound to a pound each week. When it comes to reducing weight, however, slow but steady is more effective and long-term sustainable.

7.2 Intermittent Fasting Is Not For Everyone

Not everyone should (or wants to) engage in IF. Women who are pregnant or attempting to get pregnant (long fasting periods may mess off your menstrual cycle), diabetics (blood sugar might drop too low in the absence of food), and anybody taking several prescriptions (food, or lack thereof, may impact absorption and dose), according to Kumar. Also, if you've had a background of eating disorders, adding times when you're "not permitted" to eat might set you up for a disastrous relapse.

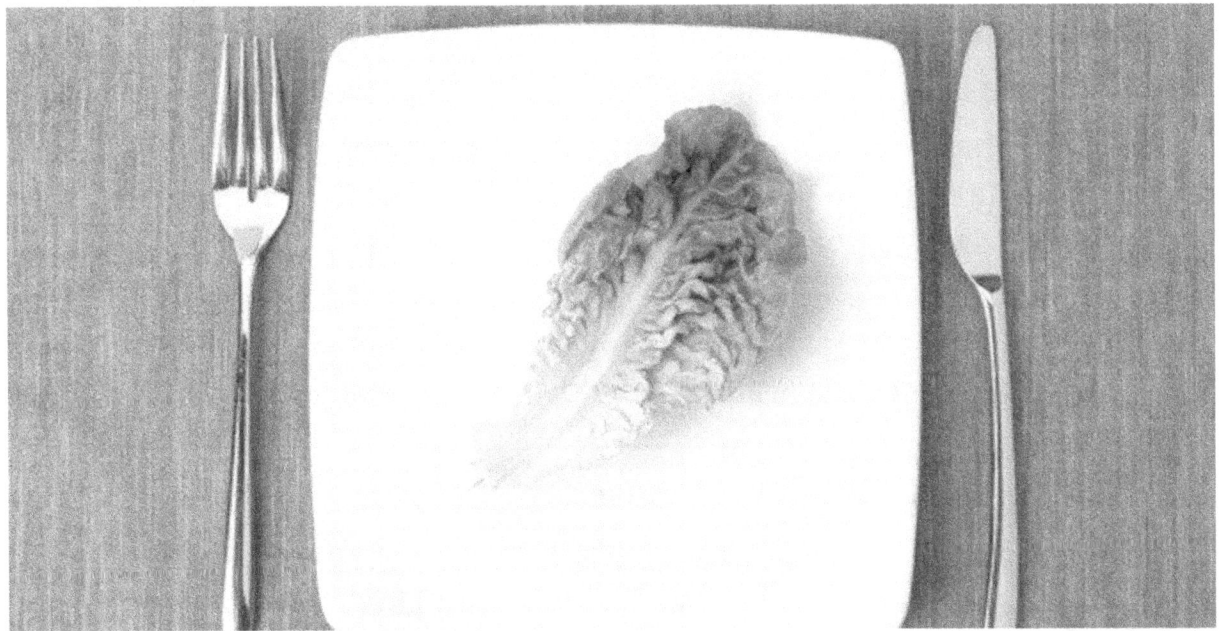

It's important to be aware that IF has certain adverse effects. Because low blood sugar may interfere with your mood, you may feel grumpy — "hanger" is real — while fasting periods. When you do eat, you must continue to consume a nutritious diet. "One thinking is that if you fasted for 2 days, it would be tough to make up your calorie deficit, but in our culture, with availability to calorie-dense foods, you could certainly manage it," Kumar adds. Concentrate on nutrient-dense foods such as fruits, vegetables, lean meats, and whole grains (Though other doctors, including Dr. Shemek, recommend combining IF with a low-carb or keto diet.). Expect poor energy, bloating, and cravings for the first several weeks while your body adapts, says Shemek.

Intermittent fasting (IF) may seem to be a complicated concept. But all it truly entails is going without food for long periods.

Why would someone want to do anything like that? According to a rising number of fitness professionals, the practice may assist individuals in losing weight and improving their health.

Intermittent fasting, on the other hand, isn't only for nutritionists. In reality, we all do it on a daily basis in some way. We don't call it that, however. It's referred to as sleeping.

That's correct. A "fasting" interval is defined as the period between your final meal at night and your first meal the following day.

(A "feeding" interval is defined as the period between your first and final meals of the day.)

That's all there is to it. So try not to become too engrossed in the terminology.

People who practice intermittent fasting merely lengthen the amount of time they go without eating in the end.

Of course, everyone is vying to be the first to "get it right." As a result, various protocols have evolved, including Eat Stop Eat, the Warrior Diet, Leangains, the 5:2 diet, and others. However, in some way or another, all of these regimens reduce the "eating" window while expanding the "not eating" window.

7.3 What Exactly Is The Purpose Of Fasting?

Intermittent fasting is not a new concept, despite the word being a recent creation. Humans have always fasted, either for a single night, a longer food shortage, or religious reasons.

What's new is that clinical studies on IF's health and lifespan advantages are now catching up.

When done correctly, data suggests that IF may help lengthen life, regulate blood glucose, lower the risk of cardiovascular disease, control blood lipids, manage body weight, help us develop (or retain) lean mass, lower the risk of cancer, and more.

Because these studies are already in their early phases, there are reasons for skepticism. However, some of the results seem to be encouraging.

That is why many fitness enthusiasts have opted to put IF to the test. They're relying on personal experimentation in the absence of reliable evidence.

7.4 Is Intermittent Fasting Right For You?

Intermittent fasting does work for some, but it may not be right for everyone.

First and foremost, intermittent fasting is not a synonym for "free ride." Skipping meals at random while consuming a high-processed food diet will not help you lose weight or improve your health.

While there is no one "correct" method to fast, every effective program will include certain dietary considerations. You must be willing to put in the effort.

Some people may find IF too difficult or inconvenient to practice. Others, on the other hand, see the hazards as far outweighing any possible advantages. In fact, some individuals may find IF to be quite harmful.

You probably like to know whether you are into that group before skipping your next meal.

Based on multiple case studies and a tiny amount of published research, here's the lowdown.

Intermittent Fasting: Green Light

In my experience, you're most likely to be successful with intermittent fasting if:

- You've previously kept track of your calorie and food consumption (e.g., you've "dieted").
- You're already a regular exerciser.
- If you're not married or don't have children,
- if you have a partner, he or she is highly supportive
- Your employment permits you to experience periods of poor performance while you adjust to a new strategy.
- You're a man

The first five characteristics will make it easier to incorporate the protocols into your daily routine, while the sixth component (being male) seems to impact outcomes.

Intermittent fasting: Yellow Light

In the meanwhile, if you satisfy the following requirements, continue with caution:

- You're married or a parent.
- You work in a client-facing or performance-oriented environment.
- You participate in sports or athletics.
- You're a woman.

Again, the first three factors following IF guidelines are much more difficult and may make them impracticable for you. Furthermore, attempting to run quickly may contradict your sport's performance objectives.

In the final problem, some researchers believe that fasting promotes sleepiness, anxiety, irregular periods, or other signs of hormone dysregulation in women.

Women, in particular, seem to perform worse than males when it comes to harsher kinds of intermittent fasting. So, if you're a woman who wants to attempt fasting, it is suggested to start slowly and gradually.

Intermittent Fasting: Red Light

As mentioned before, not everyone should use intermittent fasting, and some individuals should not do it even under certain circumstances. Don't even think about it if

- You're with child.
- You have a background of disordered eating that you've struggled with before.
- You are always under a lot of stress
- You don't get much rest.
- This is your first time on a diet and an exercise program.

Because intermittent fasting is a novel concept for you, it could seem like a magical solution for weight reduction. Instead, it would be wise to work on addressing any possible nutritional deficits before you try experimenting with fasts. Before embarking on any weight loss program, it is important to have a sound dietary foundation.

Women who are pregnant have increased energy demands; therefore, if you want to establish a family, now is not the season to fast.

If you're under constant stress and aren't getting enough sleep, you're describing the same condition. You have a stressful life, and your body needs more nurturing, not extra stress.

And if you have suffered from disordered eating as in the past, you will know that fasting might have the potential to push you down a road that may generate more difficulties for you. The answer is simple: There's no need to interfere with your health. In other words, you might attain equivalent advantages in other methods.

7.5 How To Shape Up Without Intermittent Fasting?

So you're saying intermittent fasting isn't an option for you, and you're looking for advice on how to get in shape & lose weight?

To learn the fundamentals of a healthy diet, consider studying nutrition. It's by far the finest thing you can do about your fitness and health.

Food should be cooked and eaten using entire, unprocessed ingredients. Exercise on a regular basis. Keep doing what you're doing. Finally, if you want some assistance with all of that, look for a mentor or coach.

In other words, even if you opt to go the intermittent fasting route, that final point is still significant.

While self-experimentation is beneficial, supervised experimentation is very beneficial. In particular while under the supervision of an expert coach.

Chapter 8: Health Benefits of Intermittent Fasting

While fasting has become more mainstream recently, there are several methods, some of which may vary from the standard protocols.

While there are many distinct intermittent fasting approaches, such as the 16/8 & 5:2 ways, many more fall somewhere in between these two extremes.

It seems that several research demonstrates that it may be helpful for your body and your brain.

While there are many evidence-backed health advantages associated with intermittent fasting, here are 10 more advantages:

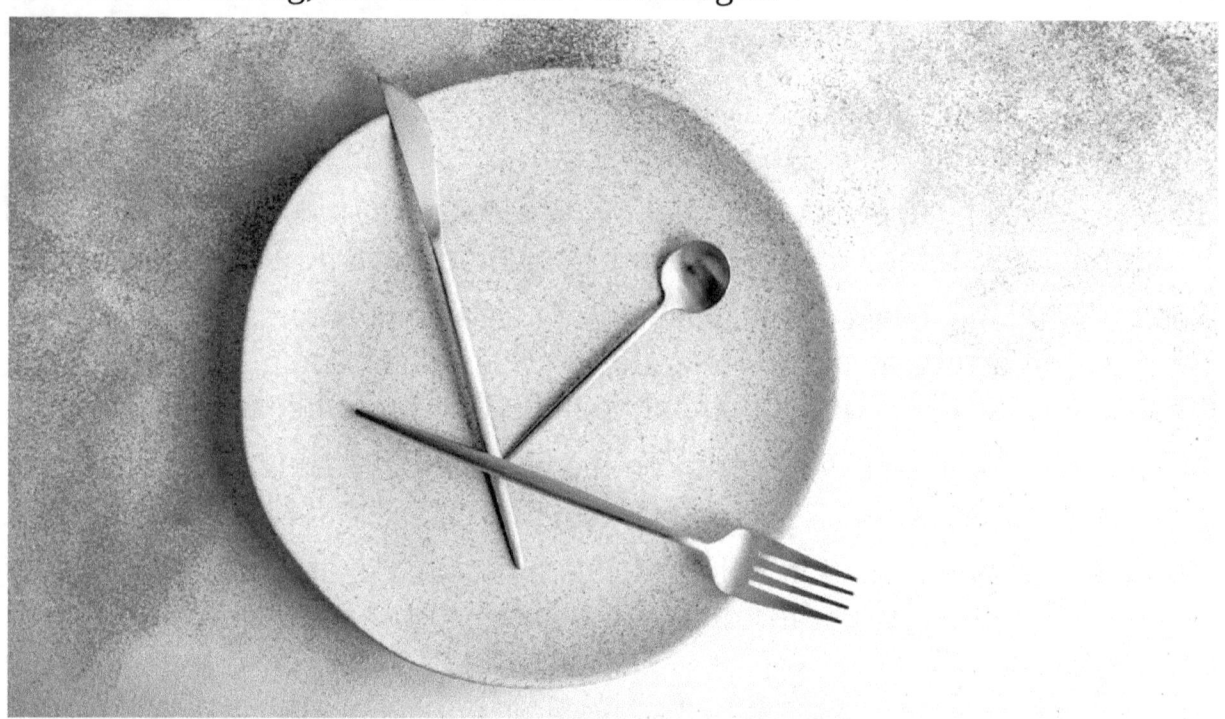

1. Change the functions of cells, genes, and hormones

Several physiological processes occur when you go without food for a period of time.

Your body, for example, alters hormone levels and makes stored body fat better accessible while also initiating crucial cellular repair activities.

Some of the physiological changes that occur while fasting is listed below:

- **Insulin levels.** The fasting insulin levels decrease dramatically, resulting in a rise in fat metabolism.
- **Human growth hormone levels.** Human growth hormone (HGH)

levels may substantially rise, resulting in increased muscle mass and muscle strength. The higher amounts of this hormone stimulate fat burning and muscle growth, and it has various additional advantages.

- **Cellular repair.** Cellular repair activities, such as removing waste material from cells, are activated by the body.
- **Gene expression.** There are several favorable alterations in many genes and molecules associated with long life and immunity against disease.

As you can see, a lot of the advantages of intermittent fasting are tied to these hormone and cell modifications, as well as gene expression.

When you abstain from food, insulin levels go down while human growth hormone increases. Additionally, your cells participate in key cellular repair activities, such as protein synthesis and alter which genes they express.

2. Help your visceral fat and lose weight

Many people who attempt intermittent fasting are motivated by their desire to reduce weight.

Generally speaking, intermittent fasting (IF) will result in you eating fewer meals.

In order to compensate for all the more calories than you'll be consuming from other meals, you'll have to reduce your caloric intake elsewhere.

In addition, intermittent fasting will help to optimize hormone activity to facilitate weight reduction.

These things, including lower insulin levels, greater HGH levels, and greater concentrations of norepinephrine (noradrenaline), all help promote the breakdown of body fat and allow it to be used as energy.

As a result, short-term fasting will help you burn more calories, which means you can make your plan work longer.

As a result, intermittent fasting acts on both sides of the equation: caloric intake and expenditure. It enhances your metabolic rate (provides more calories) while at the same time reducing the quantity of food you consume (reduces calories).

Intermittent fasting has been shown to produce weight reduction of 3 to 8 percent over the course of 3 to 24 weeks in the reviewed scientific literature. That is a significant amount.

Over the course of 6 to 24 weeks, the subjects lost anything from 4 to 7 percent of their waist circumference, thereby indicating that they shed significant amounts of visceral fat. Visceral fat is the unhealthy fat that occurs in the abdominal cavity, and it causes disease.

Another recent study has also shown that intermittent fasting leads to less muscle loss than constant calorie restriction.

However, in a randomized experiment completed in 2020, persons who used the 16/8 technique were examined. In this diet, you are on a fast for 16-hrs each day, and there is an 8-hour window in which you are permitted to eat.

Even though the participants who fasted lost much less weight than those who ate about three meals a day, the total number of calories consumed did not change. To further examine this hypothesis, the researchers also performed a body composition test on subject's in-person after some had fasted. The subjects who had fasted lost considerable amounts of lean mass. Lean muscle mass was also included.

More research is required on the relationship between intermittent fasting and muscle loss. Although it has its drawbacks, intermittent fasting can be a very strong weight reduction method.

The purpose of intermittent fasting is to consume fewer calories while slightly improving metabolism. It is a very effective weight-loss method that targets both body fat and subcutaneous fat.

3. Can reduce risk of type 2 diabetes and insulin resistance

Type 2 diabetes has been around for centuries, but it has been such a widespread diagnosis only in the last few decades.

One of the most prominent features of the condition is elevated blood sugar levels throughout the setting of insulin resistance.

The treatment of insulin resistance should reduce blood sugar levels and help prevent type 2 diabetes.

It is rather interesting. Intermittent fasting may help with insulin resistance, leading to a considerable drop in blood sugar levels.

Results from human research have shown that persons with prediabetes had lower fasting blood sugar levels after fasting for 7-12 weeks. The fasting insulin that has been lowered by between 20% - 30%.

It was shown that when mice with diabetes were exposed to intermittent fasting, they had longer life spans and reduced the chances of diabetic retinopathy. Diabetic retinopathy is a possible condition that may lead to blindness.

This suggests that intermittent fasting (IF) may be very protective for persons at higher risk of acquiring type 2 diabetes.

However, it is possible that there may be some disparities between the sexes. Another research conducted on women in 2005 found that blood sugar regulation deteriorated when intermittent fasting was done for 22 days.

Reduced insulin resistance and decreased blood sugar levels may be partly attributable to intermittent fasting in males.

4. Can reduce inflammation and oxidative stress in the body

Oxidative stress is a phase in the aging process and the development of certain chronic diseases.

Free radicals are unstable chemicals that are a part of this process. Free radicals interact with many other essential molecules, including proteins & DNA, and damage them.

Several scientific research has shown that intermittent fasting (IF) may increase the body's resilience to oxidative stress.

Research also suggests that intermittent fasting helps to reduce inflammation, which is a major contributor to a wide variety of diseases.

Scientists that performed research on intermittent fasting have shown that it may help to minimize oxidative damage & inflammation in the body. These are intended to provide advantages against aging and the development of several illnesses.

5. Maybe good for heart health

Cardiovascular disease presently claims the majority of the world's victims.

Anecdotal evidence suggests that several risk factors for heart disease (so-called "risk factors") are correlated with an increased or reduced risk of cardiovascular disease.

Various risk factors such as diabetes, heart disease, and some cancers have been proved to benefit from intermittent fasting:

- blood pressure
- blood sugar levels
- blood triglycerides
- inflammatory markers
- total & LDL (bad) cholesterol

On the other hand, a lot of this has been based on animal research.

While it is definitely important to study the impact of fasting on human heart health in greater detail, currently, there are not enough clinical trials to make recommendations.

Several studies have shown that intermittent fasting may help reduce several heart disease risk factors, such as blood pressure, triglycerides, cholesterol levels, and inflammatory markers.

6. Induces many cellular repair processes

When we are fasting, the cells in our body go through autophagy and remove cellular waste.

Breaking down and metabolizing damaged and malfunctioning proteins that pile up within cells over time is one approach to dealing with this problem.

While autophagy could help protect the body against several diseases, such as cancer and neurological disorders like Alzheimer's disease, an elevated level of autophagy might help protect the body against these diseases.

In a fasting state, a metabolic system termed autophagy is triggered, resulting in the removal of cellular waste.

7. Help reduce the risk of cancer

The uncontrolled proliferation of cells defines cancer.

Several studies have demonstrated that fasting has several favorable impacts on metabolism, including the potential to lessen cancer incidence.

Preliminary data from animal research suggests that intermittent fasting (IF) or diets that imitate intermittent fasting may help prevent cancer. Studies conducted in humans have shown consistent conclusions with those discovered in other animals, albeit further research is required.

There is some evidence to suggest that fasting may help lessen various negative effects associated with chemotherapy in humans.

In animal research, intermittent fasting has been found to help prevent cancer. On the other hand, there is little human research on intermittent fasting and cancer. An in-vitro study conducted on people shown that it may assist in decreasing the negative effects produced by chemotherapy.

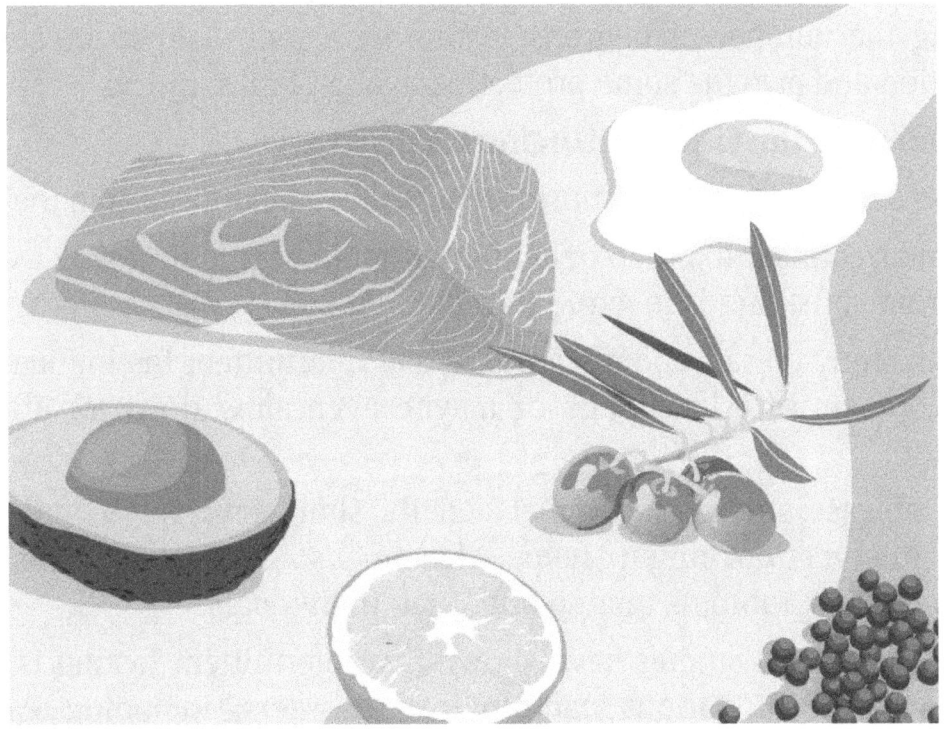

8. Has benefits for brain

Generally speaking, what is healthy for the body is beneficial for the brain.

Research suggests that intermittent fasting effectively improves many metabolic aspects that are known to be crucial for brain function.

The benefits of intermittent fasting include the reduction of:

- inflammation
- oxidative stress
- insulin resistance
- blood sugar levels

Several studies in rats and mice have shown that IF increase the number of new nerve cells, which may help may improve brain function.

The use of fasting may also lead to higher levels of a neural hormone called (BDNF) brain-derived neurotropic factor. BDNF insufficiency has been suggested to be an underlying cause of depression and other cognitive issues.

Animal studies have also demonstrated that intermittent fasting helps to protect the brain from stroke-related brain damage.

The short-term use of intermittent fasting may help to promote brain health. Increasing the number of neurons in the brain may lead to greater neuron proliferation and provide some protection against brain injury.

9. Might reduce the risk of Alzheimer's disease.

Alzheimer's disease is the most prevalent neurological disease in the world.

There is no treatment to cure Alzheimer's; therefore, the best way to keep this disease from spreading is to avoid it in the first place.

A research study on rats and mice found that intermittent fasting may prevent the development of Alzheimer's or maybe even slow down or alleviate its progression.

A series of case studies show that a daily short-term fast coupled with a lifestyle intervention might help Alzheimer's patients by considerably improving their symptoms in nine out of ten individuals.

Additionally, animal studies have shown that intermittent fasting is linked to a decreased risk of various neurological disorders, including Parkinson's disease and Huntington's disease. While more investigation in humans is required

Some evidence from animal research suggests that intermittent fasting might potentially be protective against neurodegenerative disorders such as Alzheimer's disease.

10. May extend your lifespan

One of the most intriguing applications of intermittent fasting might be the capacity to enhance life span.

Intermittent fasting enhances longevity in mice in a comparable manner as constant calorie restriction, according to research.

Fruit flies have been demonstrated to live longer after undergoing intermittent fasting.

The results of several of these investigations were extremely spectacular. In previous research, rats that fasted every second day lived 83 percent longer than rats that did not fast.

In a 2017 research, mice that were fasted every second day exhibited a 13 percent increase in their lives.

Fasting on a daily basis has also been demonstrated to benefit the health of male mice. It aided in preventing fatty liver disease & hepatocellular cancer, both of which are frequent in aged mice.

Intermittent fasting has grown increasingly fashionable among the anti-aging community, even though this has yet to be shown in people.

Logically, intermittent fasting may help you live a better and longer life, given its established advantages for metabolism and various health indicators.

Animal studies suggest that intermittent fasting may help humans to live longer.

Chapter 9: Best Foods During Intermittent Fasting

Please consult with a health expert before making any big dietary changes to ensure that it is the best alternative for you.

Intermittent fasting (IF) is creating quite a stir in the congested world of dieting, despite the word "fasting" being very ominous.

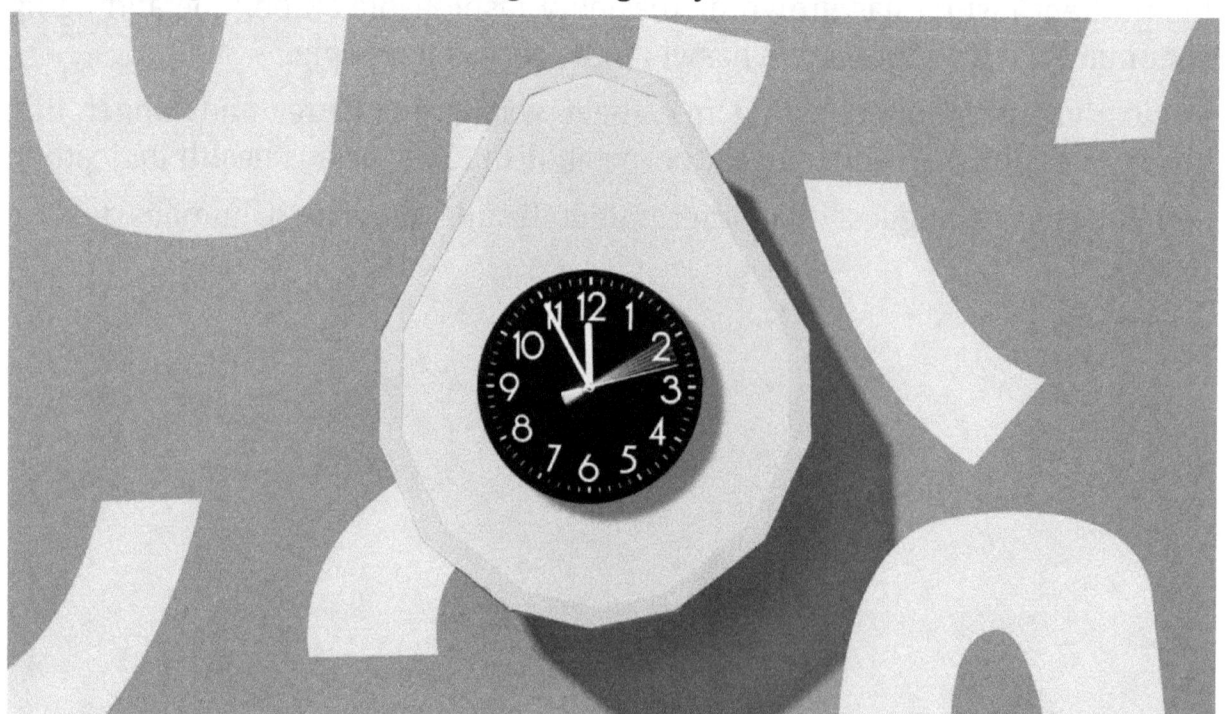

However, a substantial amount of research (however with small sample sizes) indicates that the diet may help people lose weight and control their blood sugar levels. It's no surprise that everyone and their aunt has jumped on the IF bandwagon.

Perhaps the attractiveness stems from the absence of food regulations: There are limitations on when and what you can consume, but not always on what you can consume.

What's more, there's something more to consider. Should you be breaking your fast with pints of ice cream & bags of chips? Almost certainly not. That's why we've put up a list of the greatest foods to include in your IF lifestyle.

To put it another way, if you consume a lot of the things listed below, you won't be hungry while fasting.

1. Water

It isn't exactly food, but it's crucial for making it through IF.

Water is essential for the health of almost all of your body's main organs. It would be a mistake to skip this as part of the fast. Your organs play a critical role in keeping you alive.

The quantity of water each individual should drink varies depending on their gender, height, weight, degree of exercise, and climate. The color of your urine, however, is a reliable indicator. At all times, you would like it to be light yellow.

Dehydration may induce headaches, weariness, and lightheadedness. Therefore dark yellow urine indicates that you're dehydrated. When you combine it with a lack of food, you've got yourself a formula for catastrophe - or, at the least, incredibly black urine.

If plain water doesn't appeal to you, try adding a squeeze of lemon, a few mint leaves, and cucumber slices to it.

2. Avocado

Eating the most calorie-dense fruit while attempting to lose weight may seem paradoxical. On the other hand, avocados will keep you full throughout even the most stringent fasting times because of its high unsaturated fat content.

Unsaturated fats may keep the body full even if you don't feel hungry, according to research. Your body sends out signals that it isn't going to go into emergency famine mode because it doesn't have enough nourishment. Even if you're hungry in the midst of a fasting period, unsaturated fats keep these indications continuing for longer.

Another research discovered that included half an avocado in your lunch will keep you satisfied for up to 3 hrs longer than if you don't eat the green, mushy gem.

3. Seafood and fish

There's a reason why the American Dietary Guidelines recommend two to three 4-ounce portions of fish each week.

In addition to being high in healthy fats & proteins, it is also high in vitamin D.

And if you like to eat within restricted window times, don't you want to get the most nutritious bang for your money when you do?

There are so many different methods to prepare fish that you will never run out of options.

4. Cruciferous vegetables

The f-word – fiber — is abundant in foods such as broccoli, Brussels sprouts, and cauliflower. (We understand what you're thinking, and no, that f-word does not stand for "farts.")

It's essential to consume fiber-rich meals regularly to keep you regular and ensure that your poop factory runs efficiently.

Fiber may also help you feel full, which might be beneficial if you won't eat for another 16 hours.

Cruciferous vegetables may also help you from developing cancer.

5. Potatoes

For example, in the 1990s, researchers discovered that potatoes are among the most satiating meals. In addition, a 2012 research discovered that included potatoes in a balanced diet might aid weight reduction. (Unfortunately, French fries & potato chips do not qualify.)

6. Beans & legumes

On the IF lifestyle, your favorite chili ingredient maybe your best buddy.

Food, primarily carbohydrates, provides energy for physical activities. We're not suggesting you go crazy with carbs, but including low-calorie carbohydrates like beans & legumes in your diet can't harm you. It might help you stay awake throughout your fasting period.

Furthermore, foods such as chickpeas, black beans, peas, & lentils have been demonstrated to help people lose weight even when they are not on a calorie-restricted diet.

7. Probiotics

What do the small bugs in your stomach prefer to eat the most? Consistency and variety are two things that are important to us. When they're hungry, this suggests they're not happy. And if your stomach isn't pleased, you could notice some unpleasant side effects, such as constipation.

Add probiotic-rich foods to your diets, such as kefir, kombucha, and sauerkraut, to help alleviate this discomfort.

8. Berry

These smoothie essentials are packed with minerals and vitamins. That's not even the most exciting aspect.

Persons who ate a lot of flavonoids, like those found in blueberries & strawberries, had lower BMI rises over 14 years versus people who didn't eat berries, according to 2016 research.

9. Eggs

One big egg has 6.24 grams of protein and takes just a few minutes to prepare. And, particularly when you're eating less, obtaining as much protein as necessary is vital for staying full and growing muscle.

Men who ate one egg breakfast rather than a bagel for breakfast were less hungry also ate less during the day, according to 2010 research.

To put it another way, if you're searching for something to do while you are fast, why not hard-boil a bunch of eggs? Then, when the moment is appropriate, you may consume them.

10. Nuts and seeds

Although nuts are heavier in calories than other snacks, they include something that most snack foods lack: healthy fats.

Also, don't be concerned about calories! According to 2012 research, a 1-ounce intake of almonds (about 22 nuts) has 20% fewer calories than the label indicates.

According to the research, chewing does not entirely break down the cell walls of almonds. It keeps a part of the nut intact and prevents it from being absorbed by your body during digestion. As a result, if you consume almonds, they may not make as much of a difference in your daily calorie consumption as you think.

11. Whole grains

Dieting and carbohydrate consumption seems to belong in two separate categories. It will come as a huge relief to learn that this isn't always the case. Because whole grains are high in fiber and protein, a little portion will keep you satisfied for a long time.

So go out of your comfort zone and try farro, bulgur, spelled, Kamut, millet, sorghum, or freekeh, a whole-grain utopia.

Chapter 10: Foods to Avoid while Intermittent Fasting

The problem is, having fat around your waist is entirely natural and quite common—having minimum body fat and ripped abs is rare. The problem is with the sort of fat you own: subcutaneous fat, which you can grip and touch with your fingers, is far less harmful to your health than visceral fat, which is found deep inside the abdominal cavity. Type 2 diabetes, Heart disease, and high cholesterol are just a few of the major health problems that may be caused by visceral fat.

Fortunately, you can do activities to lessen these risks (which do not entail following fad diets or engaging in negative self-talk). Exercise is critical for a long-term healthy lifestyle and fat loss (aim for at least 25 minutes of physical exercise every day, such as walking), but the foods you consume also have a role.

1. Cheese

Cheese has a high calorie and saturated fat content. It isn't to suggest that all dairy is off bounds (we don't think what to do if we couldn't have our chocolate chip ice-cream)—healthy alternatives like skim milk still provide protein and calcium to the body. Still, if you want to lose weight in your stomach, follow the French example and avoid processed, melted cheese in favor of modest quantities of additive-free cheeses.

2. Soft drinks

Artificial sugars & high-fructose corn syrup are used to sweeten soda, both of which may increase intra-abdominal fat and provide extra calories: "In general, sodas should be avoided to prevent bloating and belly obesity," Selvakumar advises. "Any residual sugar will be turned to fat and finally stored in adipose tissue."

Even if you believe you're picking the "healthier" alternative, the artificially sweet taste of diet Coke prompts your body to create insulin, which leads to increased blood sugar and a greater waist circumference.

 Avoid sugary beverages at all costs.

Substitute fruit-infused waters for sugary beverages.

3. Processed Meats

Meat may be a healthy element of your diet since it provides your body with a large amount of protein, which, though we all know, helps in the maintenance of energy levels and the development of new muscle cells. Processed meats heavy in saturated fat (that includes bacon) are not your friends when it comes to a healthy lifestyle. "It's better to avoid processed meats (such as dried meat, beef jerky, hot dogs, salami, slab bacon, sausages, and canned meats) if you're trying to reduce weight and obtain a flat tummy," says Selvakumar. "Many processed types of meat are heavy in salt, fat, & cholesterol, all of which may contribute to an increased risk of heart disease." To get your daily limit, go for plant proteins and lean meats such as grilled chicken and fish.

4. Alcohol

We hate to break it to you, but your regular happy hour could be causing more damage than good. "Alcohol has seven calories per gram, which is somewhat less than fat, which has nine calories per gram," Selvakumar explains. "Alcohol, regardless of the sort of alcoholic beverage consumed, will not assist a person in achieving a flat stomach, much alone attempting to lose weight." While wine falls into this category, it's worth noting that certain alcoholic drinks have more calories than the others (as an example, beer has a lot more calories than wine). You don't need to fully abstain from alcohol; limit yourself to one drink each sitting.

5. Salad dressings, fat-free or low in fat

You've certainly heard that eating a Mediterranean diet (one rich in lean, antioxidant-rich foods like olive oil, seafood, and leafy greens) may be beneficial to both your mind and body. On the other hand, low-fat and fat-free salad dressings may be dangerous if they include genetically modified oils that have been heated, squeezed, or refined, according to Selvakumar. Additionally, the use of high-fructose corn syrup, added sugar, and preservatives may contribute to weight gain. Instead, make your own salad dressing from scratch, in which you control all of the components. For a delightful, healthier alternative, we recommend our favorite mix. Lemon & red wine vinegar added to olive oil.

6. Fruit Juice with Added Sugar

Most store-bought fruit juices, like soda, are loaded with chemicals, sweeteners, and high-fructose corn syrup. The same may be said for smoothies purchased from a shop. According to Selvakumar, your adipose tissue (where excess sugar is converted to fat) has an infinite storage capacity, making it impossible to get a flat stomach if you consume sugary fruit juice. Try producing your own juice at home instead of going on your regular juice run. While you'll have to clean up a little more, you'll notice a difference between the freshness & your waistline will improve.

7. Refined Bread

Bread and other refined carbs should be avoided as part of a balanced diet. Inflammation & weight gain are promoted by diets high in "dense cellular carbs," according to one research. 3 Consider Ezekiel bread, flaxseed bread, oat bread, whole wheat, or rye bread as a healthy alternative to your morning bagel. You may also notice a change in your energy levels during the day, as well as a longer feeling of fullness.

Consume fibre-rich foods such as avocados, lentils, oats, and flaxseeds instead of refined bread. They'll help relax, just like bread, but they'll also help slow down the passage of food through your digestive system.

8. Cereal

Breakfast is typically referred to as the essential meal of the day, but if you consume many bowls of cereal first thing in the morning, your GI system won't have enough time to digest the food properly—not to mention that high sugar content with processed white flour might contribute to weight gain. Selvakumar suggests low-fat or skims milk for weight reduction or plant-based milk and cereals (think almond, oat & soy).

9. Salt

Although excess salt does not contribute to belly fat gain, it is a typical cause of bloating and may make you feel like you've gained a few pounds overnight.

"Unrefined salt (think sea salt & Himalayan pink salt) is the best salt to use," Selvakumar recommends. "However, you must also consider how much salt you're applying throughout the cooking process." Replace salt with fresh spices and herbs (like ginger, basil, & turmeric) to cut down on the quantity of salt used in your meals. And if you do indulge in a salty snack, be sure to drink plenty of water afterward to prevent bloating & dehydration.

10. Baked Goods

Processed baked items, according to Selvakumar, are generally high in sugar and fat, which will sabotage your efforts to get a flat tummy. If you have a sweet taste, examine the ingredient list on your product and choose low-sugar treats like vegan cakes and cupcakes. Alternatively, freeze a few grapes for a delicious "dessert" that is refreshing.

11. Fried Foods

Selvakumar, on the other hand, isn't a big lover of fried meals for a flat stomach, as we suspected. "Fried meals include more oil, fat, and cholesterol, which is counterproductive to the objective of achieving a flatter stomach," she explains. Try baking things that you would ordinarily fry in the oven—you'll use less oil and won't need to give up the crunch.

Chapter 11: Must Avoiding Mistakes While Intermittent Fasting

Intermittent fasting, a pattern of eating in which you have extended intervals of fasting and brief eating intervals, is becoming more popular. Although it's often used as a weight-loss strategy, the truth is that it isn't beneficial. On the other hand, intermittent fasting will only be successful if you maintain a healthy eating regimen throughout your feeding hours. Its means that it's almost exactly like a healthful diet for the most part. If you are experiencing difficulties, one of the most frequent intermittent fasting mistakes you may be contributing to the problem.

As someone aiming to reduce weight, you may have thought about intermittent fasting, which is one of the hottest trends in fitness and health. Many health benefits associated with intermittent fasting (e.g., weight reduction, improved body composition, lowered inflammation, reduced insulin, and more) are achievable if the process is done appropriately.

While intermittent fasting is simple in theory, it includes many more aspects than merely missing a meal or two. It is only by carefully doing things correctly that favorable outcomes are achieved.

Registered Dietitian Natalie Rizzo, RD, MS, says, "If you are only eating at particular hours of the day, then you want to make sure you're getting foods that provide nutritional value and critical nutrients at those times to provide you enough energy and critical nutrients to get you through the day." To not suffer from exhaustion, low energy, or hunger, be sure to consume a diet full of fresh fruits and vegetables.

However, if you don't fall into one of the previously mentioned categories, intermittent fasting may not be for you. It is important to note that the statement about pregnant or nursing women, individuals with a background of an eating problem, and athletes are intended for individual discretion and does not represent professional advice. The study results reveal that these groups must eat regularly and should not restrict their consumption to particular hours of the day.

Intermittent fasting is a diet regimen where you eat in cycles with controlled intervals of time during which you fast. If you are interested in doing this, you must monitor your behaviors and still profit from the advantages of the diet. Avoid these blunders when you are embarking on an intermittent fasting regimen.

1. Drastically Starting With Intermittent Fasting

To put it lightly, one of the worst blunders you can make is starting dramatically. You may leave yourself up for failure if you rush in and try to make it happen immediately in IF. While it is simple to fit three regular-sized meals or six little meals into a day, it is not simple to limit oneself to eating inside a four-hour timeframe.

Instead, ease into fasting by progressively cutting down on your calorie intake. If you are trying to stick to the 16/8 schedule, gradually expand the length of time between meals unless you can be able to work for 12 hours straight. Therefore, to narrow the frame to 8 hours, increment the daily minutes by few minutes each day until you get at the 8-hour window.

2. Not Choosing Appropriate Plan For Intermittent Fasting

You are ready to attempt Intermittent Fasting for weight reduction and have prepared by grocery shopping for meals like wild fish and free-range poultry, fresh fruits and vegetables, and whole-food side dishes like quinoa and lentils. As a result, the challenge is that you have not picked an IF strategy that would ensure long-term success. People who attend the gym 6 days a week and fast for two days should not use this regimen if they want to optimize their results.

There are many different variants of intermittent fasting, so it is vital to choose the one that is most suited to your schedule. Some require fasting each day for a particular number of hours for many days. Meanwhile, some include limiting the number of calories one may consume on particular days of the week. It is true: "If you have a job that includes many of the morning meetings, but you're not even snacking until 12 p.m., this may damage your career," adds Rizzo. You have chosen to work for your lifestyle for the intermittent fasting regimen, ensuring that it does.

To determine an ideal time to implement a new change or initiative, you should take the time to review your daily routine and determine the change or initiative that will best suit your schedule and habits.

3. Eating Too Much In Fasting Window

While people often choose Intermittent Fasting for the reduced time they have to eat, it's because the less time they have to eat, the fewer calories they consume. Still, it is expected that many individuals would consume the same amount of calories on fasting days as they would on non-fasting days. It is possible that you may not lose weight because of this.

Instead, consume less than your typical 2000 calories (or around 200 additional calories) during the period you're watching your weight. Instead, it is recommended to consume roughly 1200 to 1500 calories per day while you are on vacation from fasting. How many meals you consume will depend on the duration of the fasting frame, whether it be four, six, or eight hours. There may be instances when you have to overeat, and you are in a condition of deprivation. If this is the case, then you should revisit your approach and relax off the IF for one day to re-focus and then go back on your track.

4. Eating Wrong Foods While Fasting

Another Intermittent Fasting mistake is the tendency to overeat because of not adhering to the correct food intake. If you have the fasting window of six hours, and instead of refraining from food, you consume refined, fatty, and sugary foods during that time, you will most likely feel awful during and after.

A portion of the population chooses to feed their bodies calories with no nutritional value throughout their eating window rather than supplying their bodies with the nutrition they need. The diet of 1200 calories of Twinkies versus the diet of 1200 calories of vegetables has been proven to be equal in terms of the impact on weight. However, the diet of 1200 calories of Twinkies will make you unhealthy while the diet of 1200 calories of vegetables will not. Food is the best source of nutrients, and the most important things to take in are vitamins and minerals.

You follow a diet made up of lean proteins, healthy fats, legumes, unrefined grains, nuts, and wholesome veggies and fruits, which become your dietary staple. Furthermore, engage in between fasting, follow such clean eating habits:

- instead of going out to eat at a restaurant, cook & eat at home
- Gain an understanding of nutritional labels and familiarize yourself with foods and ingredients such as high fructose corn syrup

- & modified palm oil, which are avoided.
- Watch your sodium intake & beware of hidden sugars, especially in packaged foods.
- Instead of processed foods, try to cook as many whole foods as possible.
- Balance your plate with healthy carbs & fats, fiber, and lean proteins

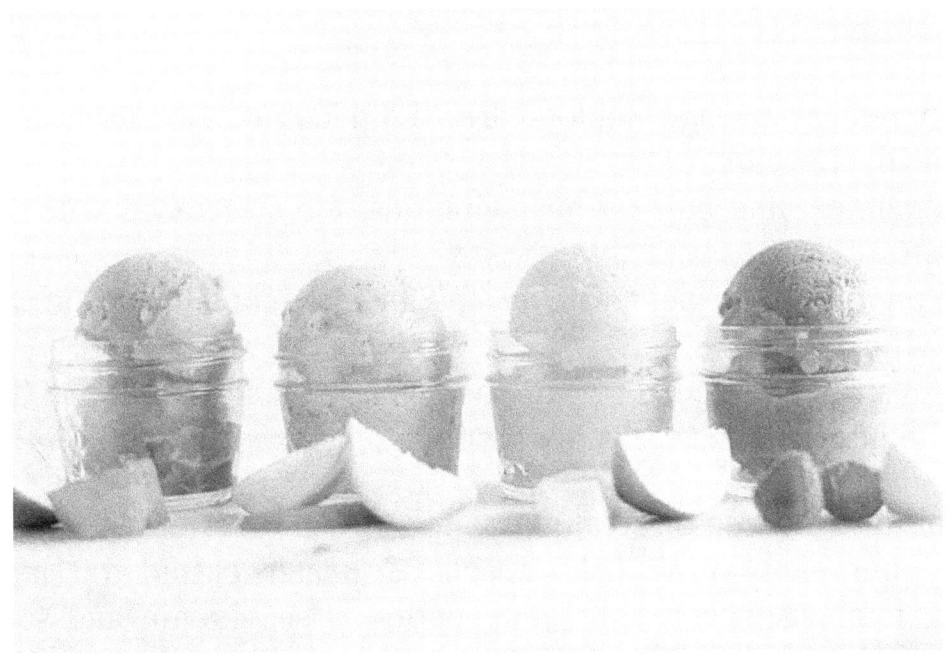

5. Restricting Calories While Fasting

It is true that there is such a thing as lowering your calories too much. To consume fewer than 1200 calories per day during your fasting window, you should eat as little as possible. Not only does it impact metabolic rate, but it may interfere with it as well. You'll gain weight if you allow your metabolism to slow too much, but you'll lose muscle if you speed it up.

Make sure to prepare your meals for the week before on the weekend so you can avoid this mistake. It provides balanced, healthful meals that are ready to be grabbed and go. You have the opportunity to have a healthy, nutritious, & caloric-correct meal when it is time to eat.

While some may go the other direction while eating, consuming adequate food is a very common practice among those who are observing their daily schedule for a specific reason. You must make sure you acquire the number of calories each day that is enough to maintain your health.

6. Unknowingly Breaking Your Intermittent Fast

If you are looking for something extra, hidden fast breakers are a good place to start. In fact, your brain responds even to a trace of sweetness, causing your body to produce insulin. Because of this, insulin is released, and this essentially breaks the fast. It is with great pleasure that we present to you the following looks at "surprise" meals, supplements, and items that may produce an insulin response:

- Ingredients such as maltodextrin and pectin that are used as additions in supplements
- Vitamins, like gummy bear vitamins, are sweetened with sugar and fats.
- You may use toothpaste & mouthwash containing the sweetener xylitol.
- Sugar may be found in pain medicines such as Advil, and hence you should take them sparingly if you're sensitive to sugar.

Do not fall into the trap of breaking your fast with intermittent fasting. After brushing your teeth using baking soda & water paste, you may use a whitening toothpaste in a non-eating period. Use vitamin and supplement labels carefully before taking supplements and vitamins.

7. Not Drinking Enough liquids When Intermittent Fasting

There are both fasting windows and eating windows during which this becomes an issue. One of the primary reasons for skipping a meal during a fast is that you tend to forget about having to drink when you are not eating. When it comes to eating, there is only one thing you want to do—that is, eat. Let me provide a suggestion that will help you with that problem. In this case, you would aim to consume 1 quart of water or 1 liter of water each day. The best time to put money into a savings account is just after you get up. Once you know how much water you're drinking, you'll always know how much more you have to drink without having to depend on memory.

While certain sections of the intermittent fasting schedule prevent you from eating, always make sure to drink water on top of everything else. It is very important to be hydrated while on an intermittent fasting diet to avoid muscular cramps, headaches and alleviate hunger pains. Therefore always stay hydrated while fasting, explains Aguirre. You may also keep hydrated by consuming water, bone broth, or bone broth-based beverages, including bone broth sparkling water, throughout your fasting window.

Undergoing intermittent fasting and getting enough water is a crucial element of IF. Keep this in mind: The amount of water taken in is equal to the amount of water lost through perspiration. The source of this, and the impact that it has, is that side effects may easily derail you if you aren't attentive. In addition to headaches, muscular cramps, and extreme sensations of hunger, if you do not keep yourself properly hydrated, dehydration will lead to the appearance of headaches, muscular cramps, and severe hunger feelings.

To prevent this problem and to prevent having irritating symptoms like cramps and headaches, incorporate the following in your daily routine:

- Water
- Water & 1-2 tbsp. apple cider vinegar (can even curb the hunger)
- Black coffee
- Herbal, black, oolong, or green tea

8. Not Exercising while Intermittent Fasting

Some individuals believe they cannot exercise while they are doing intermittent fasting, but it is the perfect condition in reality. Exercise can help you use up the fat you've accumulated. Another bonus is that Human Growth Hormone is also raised as you exercise, allowing you to gain muscle. If you know what you're doing, there are things you can do to get the most out of your exercises.

Remember the following guidelines if you want to receive the finest outcomes from your efforts:

- As far as eating concerns, try to time your exercises within the eating intervals and then have good carbohydrates & proteins within 30 minutes after your activity.
- If the workout is strenuous, ensure that you have had enough carbohydrates prior so that your glycogen reserves are sufficient
- always use the fasting approach when you are planning your workout; do not schedule an intense activity on the same day if you

are conducting a 24-hour fast
- Make sure to stay hydrated throughout the fast and particularly throughout your exercise.
- Beware of fatigue and light-headedness: if you feel you are too weak or light-headed, you should stop the exercise and give your body a rest.

9. An Unrealistic Expectation Of Yourself If You Give Up When You Slip On Intermittent Fasting

One mistake does not make a person worthless. It will happen that you will have a day or two when the IF regimen is extremely challenging, and you are not certain you can do it. You may need to take breaks if you feel overwhelmed, but it's very OK to do so. It's OK to give yourself one day to regroup before trying again. It is recommended that you try to stay on such a healthy eating track, but make allowances for occasional indulgences like a good protein smoothie or a dish of beef and broccoli and resume your normal eating habits the following day.

One of the major mistakes many people make while using intermittent fasting is to assume that it is their new whole life. Put this in your healthy living strategy: Do a component of your healthy lifestyle, and make sure you're not neglecting other things essential to you. Include enjoying a book, working out, spending time with loved ones, and eating as healthily as possible. You can achieve your goals by working hard, so it's all a part of getting to your best.

The idea is that some individuals work out when they're hungry but don't want to do something too challenging, like anything intense, since they feel it would be a problem. You should not exercise without having something to fuel your system, and it might be unhealthy to do so, advises Registered Dietitian Nicole Hinckley, LD. Be sure to have a bit before you exercise, or have a bar in the bag to make sure you feel sated before you begin.

To get the same effect of a weight-bearing exercise without putting stress on your joints, Aaptiv has yoga routines that can be done via the app.

10. Switching Fasting Times in Last Minute

It causes you to skip a party, which causes you to discover the window of time that you're focusing on your eating. There's no way to know for sure whether you could succeed if you tried to alter your schedules around, but it's going to be much tougher to stay on the diet if you do. Make an effort to check your calendar a few days in advance though you can prepare better for certain eating windows, but don't get ahead of yourself; leave yourself a week or two to change schedules.

11. Giving Up

Many individuals give up too soon when they attempt to use intermittent fasting. It takes time to expand. You will start to notice the advantages that this provides for you.

12. Binge Eating

Binge eating is something that happens when you have a restricted eating window. Regardless of how you choose to break it down, calories are always there. It is impossible to lose weight if you consume more than 10,000 calories throughout your eating window; sorry, but it's simply not possible. Neither physically nor mentally is it likely to be good for you. When individuals say "eat anything you want", they're only talking about being within specified health boundaries.

13. Making Dangerous Decisions

There are several errors in practice that people make. Some people choose strange and potentially dangerous alternatives. It happens, for example, because they believe that their fasting is effective, so they want to add one more day or make their eating window shorter. Instead, concentrate on your health.

14. Drinking Tea and Coffee

People who play games and enjoy IF sometimes say it's all right to drink coffee and tea while fasting. However, if you want to see real health benefits to the body, you won't follow through with it. Coffee is wonderful, but not only does it activate your liver, but even herbal teas (or all teas, for that matter) have the same effect. With this in mind, IF is designed to provide your body with a well-deserved break, particularly your liver. There is only one thing you should drink throughout your fasting periods, and that is water. If you are certain that you will be able to eat & drink soon, it is simple to just drink water.

15. Eating Whatever You Want

You will never really restrain yourself from overeating if you eat at certain times of the day rather than limiting your consumption to just one meal or a certain time frame. Intermittent fasting may initially positively affect your weight and health, but the impact may go rapidly if you eat the incorrect sorts of food.

Dr. Rizzo explains, "If your daily food intake consists mostly of fried foods & sweets, you will lose out on key nutrients and will end up feeling gross." Even while you no longer need to get your quota of fruits, healthy fats, whole grains, vegetables, and lean proteins during intermittent fasting, you must still acquire the foods mentioned earlier to maintain your normal caloric intake.

16. Not Eating Enough Food

Intermittent fasting is often used to help people lose weight, and thus you may feel tempted to limit calories while you're fasting. However, that is not the point, Rizzo points out. Instead of concentrating on certain eating and fasting times, you should instead aim to reduce weight. "Therefore, there is no need to restrict your caloric intake."

Instead of restricting calories, focus on filling your diet with healthy meals throughout your eating window. Restricting food intake can lead to weight loss, but your body still requires adequate food to maintain proper organ function and to remain alert, according to registered dietitian and dietetic internship program director Carol Aguirre MS, RD/LDN.

17. Feeling Guilty When You Eat Outside Your Frame

If you are hungry and believe you need food, be attentive to your body's signals. According to Rizzo, "It is OK to satisfy your hunger." "To have a good relationship with food, you must ignore your hunger cues." To avoid getting oneself into a bad mood due to hunger, always remember to allow yourself to eat whenever you're hungry. As it is said before, starving is not the objective of intermittent fasting. Therefore, if you are suffering from any unpleasant symptoms, be sure to take care of yourself.

Chapter 12: Intermittent Fasting Tips For Success

While several fasting or intermittent plans may work for you, there are several schedules to pick from that are best suited to your lifestyle. These are a few excellent suggestions:

- **The 16/8 diet**: Eat anything you want for eight hours each day and restrict your food intake to a few meals for the remaining four hours.
- **The 5:2 diet**: Consume your ordinary, everyday calorie intake five days a week, and cut down on calories to about half on the other two days. The calorie levels that are saved on these "fasting" days sometimes amount to 500 for women.
- The 14:10 diet: Somewhat similar to the 16:8 approach, since you will only be fasting for 14 hours each day and then eating for 10, therefore making it simpler to follow but not always simpler to drop weight.

If you are fasting, these are the most important guidelines to follow to effectively and properly do an intermittent fast.

1. Take It Easy! Its Your New Eating Plan

Although the desire to start a new eating habit (during the first phase of excitement) is great, doing so may be challenging and may lead to even more hunger and discomfort, as explained by Michal Hertz, a dietitian from New York City. Instead, she proposes to begin gently, for example, by using IF for two to three days each week during the first week and then increased each week progressively. Taking things slowly is a terrific way to be safe when fasting, but it's also fantastic advice for life.

2. Being Aware Of The Distinction Between Hunger And A Desire To Eat Is Important.

The first time you hear your stomach rumble, it seems as if you will have to endure a certain number of additional hours before you get a meal. Pay attention to that hungry signal. You may determine if the hunger is boredom versus true hunger by asking yourself whether you have enough to eat, suggests Eliza Savage, a registered dietitian of Middleburg Nutrition in Brooklyn. "If you are bored, you can use something else to entertain yourself." You may want to start by clearing up your inbox to make space for new emails.

However, if you're hungry but don't feel weak or dizzy (both of which are indicators that you should cease fasting immediately), you can sip a warm herbal tea since peppermint is believed to lower your appetite. Drink water to fill your stomach till your next meal, according to Savage.

In this case, if you've been practicing intermittent fasting for some time and you still experience intense hunger between cycles, then you need to consider anything. A new option that you have is to increase the nutrient- or calorie-dense items you are eating throughout your eight-hour period, or you may want to rethink if this is the right approach for you, Hertz advises. Adding healthy fats, such as avocado, coconut & olive oils, nut butter, and proteins at the start of meals will help you feel more pleased and full during the meal and throughout the day.

3. Eat When Necessary.

To be safe, though, listen to your body if you experience acute lightheadedness. There's a chance your body is trying to tell something to you. You may have low blood sugar, and you should eat something. Repeat after me: It's alright to eat anything if you have low blood sugar.

Noting that for fasting to be successful, one must remove all food, whether tiny or large, as a caution against beating oneself up if one consumes a tiny or large mouthful. Generally speaking, your best bet is that instead of reaching for high-carb snacks, it is a good idea to go for protein-rich snacks like the few cuts of turkey breast or about one-two hard-boiled eggs since they aid in keeping the body in a ketogenic (fat-burning) state, advises the nutritionist. If you're feeling up to it, you may return fasting, which is, of course.

4. Hydrate, Hydrate, Hydrate.

Although it is discouraged during periods of fasting, you are permitted to consume water and other beverages like coffee and tea (without milk) when doing so isn't going to interfere with your hydration goals.

She suggests creating reminders throughout the day, especially during fasting times, to make sure you drink lots of liquids. To help you estimate how much fluid you should be getting each day, we have Hertz and Savage both suggesting between two and three liters each day.

5. Break Your Fast Steadily And Slowly.

A few hours of food-free eating might make you feel like it's a human vacuum with a desperate want to eat everything on your plate. Although eating in a short amount of time is not recommended for your health or your waistline, some data support this theory. Instead, you like to chew thoroughly and eat slowly to give your digestive system the time it needs to thoroughly process the meal, Savage advises. The outcome of this is that you will be more informed of your fullness, which will help you avoid unnecessary weight gain.

6. Avoid Overeating.

Alternatively, because you've ended your fast, you shouldn't indulge, especially when it comes to food. It is not only possible to eat too much and be uncomfortable and bloated, but it is also possible to throw off the weight reduction objectives that drove you to IF in the top place. It's not always how much food is on your plate, which may help you feel full for longer; what is on the plate might impact that.

7. Maintain Balanced Meals.

To achieve long-term weight loss and keep yourself away from falling into a severe calorie deficiency, it is important to have a blend of healthy fats, fiber, protein, and carbohydrates in your daily diet. An excellent example, in Savage's opinion? This meal includes grilled chicken (you want around 4 to 6 oz. of protein), served with half of the sweet potato, plus sautéed spinach with garlic & olive oil.

When it concerns fruits, you like to go for those with a low glycemic index, which has slower digestion, absorption, and metabolism, leading to a slower and more sustained increase in blood glucose. Having consistent, normal blood sugar levels helps you avoid cravings, so blood sugar levels are critical when it comes to effectively losing weight.

8. Play With Different Time Frames.

While Hertz mostly advises the 16:8, she encourages customers to take note of their everyday routines and choose the fasting approach that fits their lifestyle.

For example, if you are an early riser, Hertz proposes that you eat in the morning from 10 a.m. - 6 p.m. and then abstain from food until the next morning from 10 a.m. to 6 p.m. For the record, it's crucial to note that the great thing about IF is that it's quite easy to alter and suit your schedule.

In addition, according to Savage, the only other alternative is to end your fast earlier and progressively increase your fasting strength by having breakfast later each day. All of us naturally go without food for a day every week, so it is reasonable to practice shutting off the kitchen each morning before you go to bed. A simple but helpful example is "close" your kitchen at 9 p.m., then don't eat again till breakfast at 8 a.m. It's very normal to go without food for 11 hours. Yes, if you would like, you may slowly change such timings (e.g., kitchen shuts at 8 p.m., then breakfast at 9 a.m.) if necessary.

9. Listen To Your Body.

It is really important. Keep your eyes open at all times for signs such as dizziness, weariness, unusual irritability, headache, anxiety, and a lack of concentration. If you encounter any of these symptoms, you should consider breaking your fast. Savage suggests that the body is into hunger mode and will want nutrition, "This may be all the indications that the body needs sustenance to be revitalized," she states. When you feel colder than usual, you are supposed to quit fasting, and if you begin to feel progressively colder, you should immediately cease.

It should be noted, however, that being patient is essential. Your body may probably need time to adjust to fasting, or you may experience a lack of energy and an increase in your appetite until you become acclimated to it. Do not get worked up if you experience these (far less severe) symptoms after a week or so. It may continue for some time, so if you suffer symptoms like the ones listed above, such as dizziness, Savage advises quitting the diet and trying something different to help you reach your objectives.

Chapter 13: Healthy Recipes For Intermittent Faster

Intermittent fasting (IF) is a healthy method of increasing energy and improving mental clarity while also losing weight.

While being strict about one's diet is a vital component of this process, what you consume in between meals is just as significant. Here are some meals and drinks that you should include in your IF regime.

While fasting is often defined as abstinence from eating for a set duration, it is defined as an alternate condition. In many cultures, fasting has been practiced for centuries for both spiritual and cultural objectives and only recently has a cultural update in emphasis taken place, and now it is employed for the goal of overall health.

13.1 Best Food To Break An Intermittent Fast

When it comes to BulletProof Coffee and fasting, it is important to remember several additional items you will want to consume throughout your intermittent fasting time.

Because you have to take all of your nutrients during "feeding" periods, maximizing the advantages of IF means that you should take in as much energy-dense food as possible.

If you fill your diet with whole foods, such as whole grains, fruits, and vegetables, your body will be able to absorb nutrients much more effectively, and you will be able to fast for longer periods.

Break your fast with lean proteins.

It's better to take your favorite types of protein to eat after a long period of fasting include chicken, beef, pig, turkey, eggs and seafood.

Breaking your fast with healthy fats.
While it is discussed before that Bulletproof Coffee, grass-fed butter, seeds, nut butter, nuts, olive oil, coconut oil & avocados are all fantastic healthy-fat alternatives to consume to break your fast.

Eat all the veggies that you want.
It is something you already know, but breaking your fast with a substantial serving of vegetables is always a good choice.

To-go smoothies, such as the Blueberry Muffin Smoothie or the Green

Pineapple Smoothie, may save you time in the mornings when you don't have time to cook a full meal. The lettuce and spinach both provide quite a bit of green, yet they are packed with nutrients.

Eat one plateful of fruit.

Either fresh or frozen, a dish of fruit is a pleasant way to get the micronutrients you need. To maintain healthy blood sugar levels, it is recommended that individuals eat just one serving of it.

Fruits and juices that come in cans or glass bottles tend to be highly concentrated sources of sugar, so it's better to avoid them.

Complex Carbohydrates to eat.

You may also get white potatoes, sweet potatoes, quinoa, rice, oats, and other nutritious grains.

In general, it is better to avoid high-sugar meals and go for healthy proteins & fats in place of sugary carbohydrates while breaking your fast. Or, like as it is said before, forgo the bowl of cereal or have eggs or an omelet instead.

13.2 Delicious and Healthy Recipes

Here are some simple, tasty meal ideas full of nutrients and don't need any difficult preparations.

1. Savory Oats Bowl and Roasted Veggies

Wonderful if you're looking for the first meal as breakfast. Savory, herb-flecked oats are laden with roasted vegetables and a fried egg, and as a result, they are a great way to eat nutritious and filling food for those who have just finished a fast.

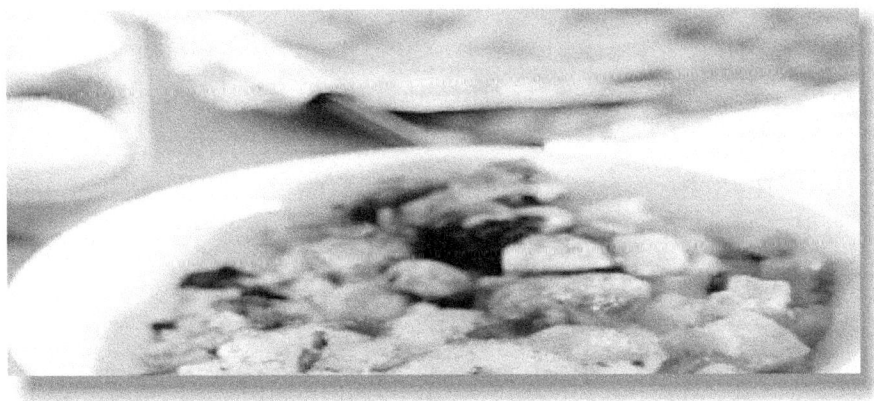

Ingredients

- 8 oz. Brussels sprouts, halved
- 16 oz. bag cubed butternut squash
- 1 tbsp. olive oil
- 1 tsp. salt, divided
- 1 tsp. black pepper, divided
- 1 tbsp. butter
- ½ cup of onion, coarsely chopped
- 2 cups of water
- 2 cups of Quaker Old Fashioned Oats
- 4 eggs
- ½ cup of shredded Sharp Cheddar cheese
- 2 strips cooked, crumbled, turkey bacon

Instructions

1. Preheat the oven to 400F. Position a large baking sheet lined with paper on top of the food.
2. In a large bowl, add the butternut squash, chopped onion, olive oil, Brussels sprouts, ½ tsp. salt, and ½ tsp. black pepper, and toss to blend. Transfer the mixture to a baking sheet and bake in the oven until the vegetables are tender about 15 minutes.
3. To get the best possible result, cook for around 20 to 22 minutes, or until the vegetables are soft and golden brown.
4. When the vegetables in the large pot are roasted in a separate saucepan, melt the butter on medium heat. Toast the oats for 30 seconds, then add them to the skillet. Next, add the water to the pan and simmer gently. Add a little water to the oatmeal, bring it to a boil, and then turn heat to low and cook for 8 - 10 mines until the oats form a thick consistency. Then stir in the shredded cheese and season with the remaining pepper and salt.
5. Place a big non-stick pan in the oven and set the temperature to the desired doneness, cooking eggs sunny-side up.
6. Soak, chop, mix oats, and any other vegetables you may choose with an egg, and then add bacon bits to the top.

2. Mediterranean Chicken Farro Bowls

Mediterranean Farro Bowls are hearty and refreshing, Farro is a high-protein and fiber-rich food, and the grilled chicken and Tzatziki sauce adds to its nutritional benefits.

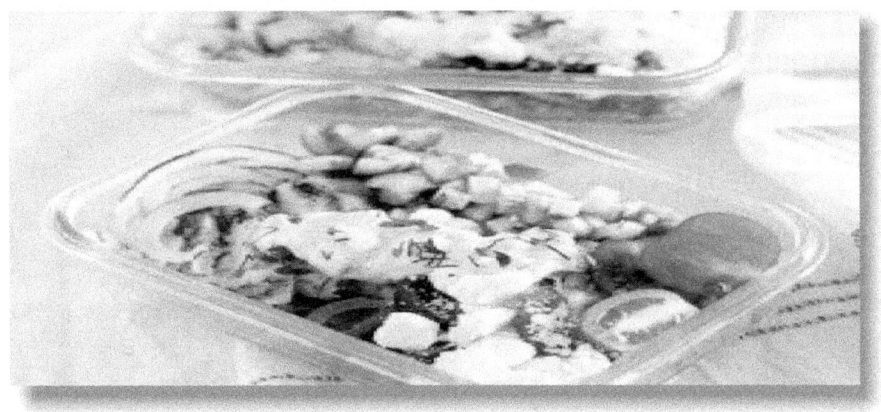

Ingredients

For The Bowls

- 1 cup of cooked Farro
- 3 cups of water or stock
- 1 lb. boneless skinless chicken breasts
- 1/2 tsp. salt
- 3 tbsps. olive oil
- 2 tbsps. lemon juice
- Zest of 1 lemon
- 2 cloves garlic, grated
- 1/2 tsp. kosher salt
- 1 tsp. dried oregano
- 1/4 tsp. black pepper
- 1 pint of cherry halved tomatoes
- 1 tbsp. olive oil
- 2 cups of chopped cucumber
- 1 cup of kalamata olives, pitted & sliced
- 1/2 sliced red onion
- Lemon wedges, for serving
- 1 cup of tzatziki sauce
- 1/2 cup of crumbled feta cheese
- Fresh dill & parsley, optional for garnish

Tzatziki Sauce

- 1 cucumber
- 1 cup plain yogurt
- 1 garlic clove
- 1/4 tsp. dried dill
- 1/2 tsp. salt

- 1/2 tsp. lemon juice

Instructions

For The Bowls

1. Add salt to a saucepan of farro, cover it, and then add enough water and stock to cover it. Bring it to a boil; then, decrease the heat to medium-low & simmer for 30 minutes. Pour off any remaining water.
2. For chicken, add one or two dozen chicken breasts into a gallon zip bag, then drizzle with olive oil, zest of one lemon, juice of two lemons, minced garlic, dried oregano, salt, and black pepper. Let it marinate for at least 4 hrs. or overnight.
3. In a large pan, heat olive oil over med-high, add the chicken breasts, and cook for 8 minutes, flipping the breasts halfway through cooking. Continue to cook for an additional 5 to 7 minutes till the internal temperature reaches 165. Discard marinade.
4. Take chicken out of the pan and wait for 5 minutes before slicing.
5. The Greek bowls, which may be found in a number of sizes, maybe assembled by adding a bed of farro in the bottom of the bowl or meal prep box. To finish, top with sliced chicken, cucumber, olives, red onion, tomatoes, tzatziki sauce & feta cheese. Add some dill and parsley to each dish, and with lemon wedges, serve.

Tzatziki Sauce

1. Strain the liquid into a large bowl lined with a mesh strainer, then transfer the liquid to a separate paper towel.
2. Squeeze the excess moisture out of the cucumber & garlic clove using a cheese grater. Then place the mixture in the strainer to remove the additional liquid.
3. Mix the shredded cucumber, yoghurt, salt, lemon juice, garlic, and dill in a medium bowl. Stir until well combined and chill for one hour before serving.

3. Shrimp and Cauliflower Fried Rice

A great low-carb dish owing to cauliflower rice, fried rice has a high protein count and a better alternative to take-out than conventional Chinese food without the accompanying crash in energy.

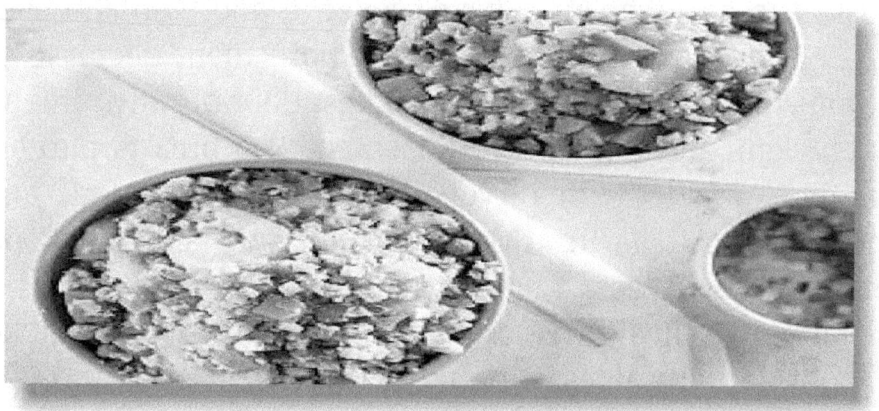

Ingredients

- 1 head of cauliflower (large) or, 6 cups of cauliflower rice
- ¼ cup of Reduced Sodium Tamari, soy sauce or Coconut Amino
- 1 Tbsp. honey
- ½ tsp. of grated fresh ginger or, ground ginger ⅛ tsp.
- 1 tbsp. sesame oil
- Pinch red pepper flakes
- 1 bunch green onions, whites separated from greens, chopped
- 3 eggs, beaten
- ½ cup of frozen peas
- ½ cup of carrots, cubed
- ½ lb. shrimp, peeled & deveined, thawed,

Instructions

1. Cut the cauliflower into small pieces and put it in a food processor. To finely chop, pulsate until the mixture looks like cooked rice, and put aside.
2. To a small bowl, add San-J Tamari, honey, ginger & red pepper

flakes. Whisk together until the sauce is slightly thickened.
3. Add sesame oil to a large skillet over medium-high heat, and let it heat up. Cook the white portion of the onions for approximately a minute after the onions have been added to the skillet. Frozen peas & carrots should be added, and the dish should be cooked until heated through for around two minutes. Place your vegetables on one side of the pan, and then add the beaten eggs to the other side. To cook eggs on the side of the pan, add the eggs to the pan and heat them around the pan until the eggs are cooked through. Stir in the shrimp, and simmer for approximately 2 minutes until the shrimp have gone pink.
4. Rice the cauliflower and add it to the mixture to combine. After the Tamari sauce mixture has been poured over the top, be sure to spread it out evenly so it can begin to cook. The sauce should have the "al dente" texture of just-cooked cauliflower when it has through cooking. Turn off the heat, put in some green onions, and cover for just a minute to let the onions soften.

4. Greens Kale Salad with Ginger Sesame Dressing

Awesome kale salad with ginger sesame dressing is one that you will come to time and time again. This Asian-inspired salad is one of the greatest you will ever prepare.

Ingredients

For the Salad

- 5 cups chopped kale (like 1 large head)
- ¼ cup of sunflower seeds
- 1 cup of shredded carrots
- ½ cup of thinly sliced red onion
- 2 cups of red cabbage, shredded
- 1 cup of shelled edamame, thawed

For the Ginger Sesame Dressing

- ½ cup of rice vinegar
- ¼ cup of soy sauce

- 3 tbsps. of sesame seeds
- 1 tbsp. of brown sugar
- 1 ½ tsps. of sesame oil
- 2 tsps. of freshly grated ginger
- 1 clove of grated garlic

Instructions

For Kale Salad

1. Put shredded red cabbage, shredded carrots, shredded kale, shelled edamame, chopped red onion, and sunflower seeds in a large bowl. Drizzle with a sesame ginger dressing to serve.

For Ginger Sesame Dressing

1. Add the salad dressing ingredients to a large bowl and mix them together. Transfer to a jar and store it in the refrigerator for up to one week.

5. Bacon & Spinach Mini Quiches

If you're in the mood for something substantial, try grain-free spinach and bacon quiches. They make a great meal or make a great lunch if you pack them inside a lunchbox the next day.

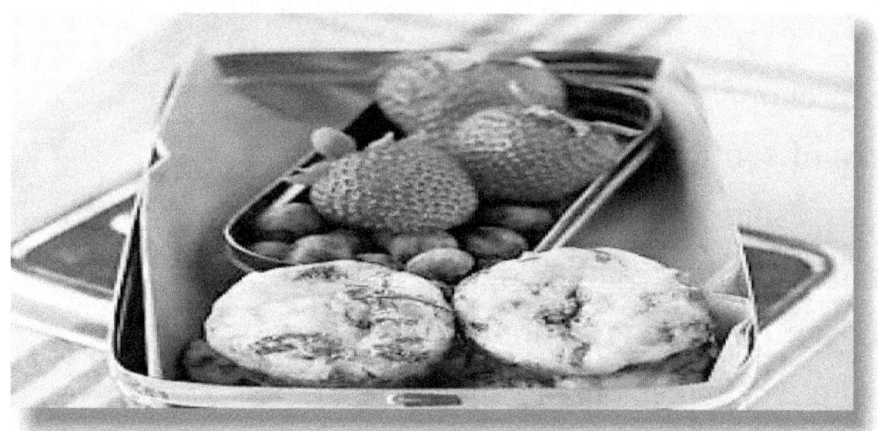

Ingredients

- 3 tbsps. milk

- 6 eggs
- ¾ cup of spinach finely chopped
- Dash of pepper
- 1 cup of cheddar shredded cheese
- 4 strips of bacon, chopped & cooked

Instructions

1. Preheat the oven to 350F and oil a 24-mini muffin pan.
2. Whisk together the eggs and milk in a large bowl. Dice up some spinach, shred some cheddar, and chopped up some bacon. Then, include pepper. Also, give it a swift stir to blend all the ingredients.
3. Distribute the egg mixture equally into the muffin pan cups.
4. Bake in preheated oven for 14 to 18 minutes.
5. To make sure that the tiny quiches have sufficiently cooled in the pan, you may either use a tiny knife or spatula to remove them.

6. Pizza Mini Quiches (Egg Cups)

Egg cups, which are filled with eggs, cheese, milk, and any of your preferred add-ins, are a fantastic source of fat and protein that will keep everyone satiated for a longer period. These egg cups are prepared with eggs, cheese, milk, and other add-ins you choose and include healthy fats and protein that will keep the whole family satiated and full for longer.

Ingredients

- 3 tbsps. milk
- 1 cup of shredded mozzarella
- 6 eggs
- ½ cup of pepperoni slices

Instructions

1. Preheat the oven to 350 ° and oil the tiny muffin pan.
2. Whisk together the eggs and milk in a large bowl. Throw in pizza toppings & shredded cheese. The key to successful mixing is to thoroughly blend all of the components.
3. Distribute the egg mixture equally into the muffin pan cups. Bake for 15 to 18 minutes.
4. Mini quiches should be allowed to cool in the pan before gently removed using a little knife or spatula.

7. Chocolate Keto Spicy Fat Bombs

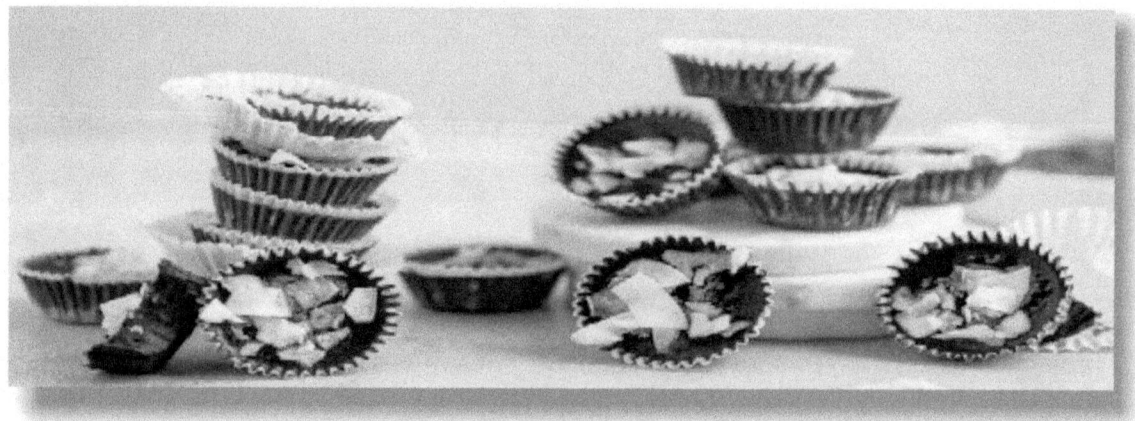

Ingredients

- 2/3 cup of smooth peanut butter
- 2/3 cup of coconut oil
- 1/2 cup of dark cocoa
- 4 packets of stevia
- 1/2 cup of toasted coconut flakes
- 1 tbsp. of ground cinnamon
- 1/4 tsp. of kosher salt
- 1/4 tsp. of cayenne (to taste)

Directions

1. Mix coconut oil, peanut butter & cocoa powder, set up a double boiler with a heating water pot. Heat the mixture until melted & smooth.
2. Stevia, cinnamon, & salt should be added and stirred to mix.
3. Divide the mixture evenly among silicone mini muffin trays. Or line a small muffin tray with liners and fill the tins up to the top with the mixture.
4. To serve, top with coconut & cayenne and place in the freezer for 30 minutes to set before slicing.

8. Cheesy Chicken Salad (Veggie Packed)

Ingredients

- 1 cup of cooked skinless boneless cubed chicken breast
- 1/4 cup of carrot, shaved into ribbons
- 1/4 cup of finely chopped celery
- 1/2 cup of Baby Spinach, chopped roughly
- 2 1/2 tbsps. mayonnaise fat-free
- 2 tbsps. of sour cream nonfat
- 1/8 tsp. of dried parsley
- 2 tsps. of Dijon mustard
- 1/4 cup of reduced-fat sharp shredded cheddar cheese

Directions

1. Add all of the ingredients to a bowl and stir well to thoroughly coat the items with the mayonnaise mixture.
2. Refrigerate for at least 35 minutes before serving, but you could even make it the night before.

9. Vegan Fried-Fish Tacos

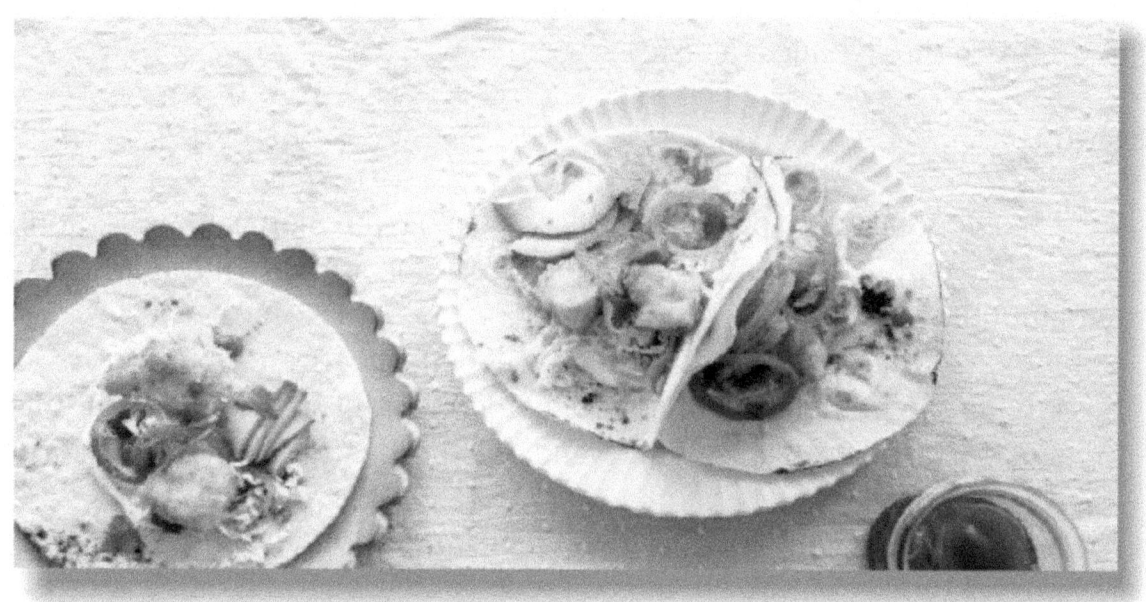

Ingredients

- 2 cups of panko breadcrumbs
- 14 oz. of silken tofu
- 1/2 cup of plain flour
- 8 small tortillas
- 1/2 tsp. of salt
- 1 tsp. of smoked paprika
- 1/2 tsp. of cayenne pepper
- vegetable oil
- 1 tsp. of ground cumin
- 1 ripe avocado
- 1/2 cup of non-dairy milk
- 1/4 finely shredded head cabbage
- vegan mayonnaise, to serve

Pickled Onion

- 1 peeled red onion, finely sliced
- 1 tsp. of salt
- ¼ cup of apple cider vinegar
- 1 tbsp. of sugar

Directions

1. The excess moisture on the tofu may be removed by patting the tofu with a few pieces of kitchen roll. Instead of slicing the tofu into perfect 1-inch cubes, use a knife to cut it into roughly 1-inch pieces.
2. Instead of slicing the tofu into perfect 1-inch cubes, use a knife to cut it into roughly 1-inch pieces.
3. Using one broad, shallow dish, place the breadcrumbs in it.
4. Sprinkle the flour, smoked paprika, cayenne, cumin, and salt into another large, shallow bowl and whisk the ingredients together.
5. To be specific, place the milk into the third wide shallow bowl.
6. Once the tofu has been sliced, lightly sprinkle it with flour, milk, and breadcrumbs. Arrange it on a baking sheet and into the oven for about 10 minutes.
7. Pour vegetable oil into a deep frying pan, the depth of which is half an inch. Pour the oil into a medium-sized pot over medium heat and let it heat up. Add a breadcrumb to the oil if it starts to bubble and brown, then the oil is ready. Fry the tofu pieces in a pan until golden below, then turn and cook on the other side to give it an even coating of golden brown. Line a baking sheet with kitchen roll and remove to drain. For the remaining tofu, repeat the same steps.

For the pickled onion:

1. Add the apple cider vinegar, salt, and sugar to a small saucepan and heat them until they begin to steam. Add the sliced red onion to a bowl or glass jar, then pour hot vinegar over it. Allow the dough to remain for at least 35 minutes to allow it to soften and become pink.
2. Serve the fried hot tofu in warmed tortillas, pickled onion, mayo, a smear of vegan avocado, and shredded cabbage.

10. Supper Club Tilapia Parmesan

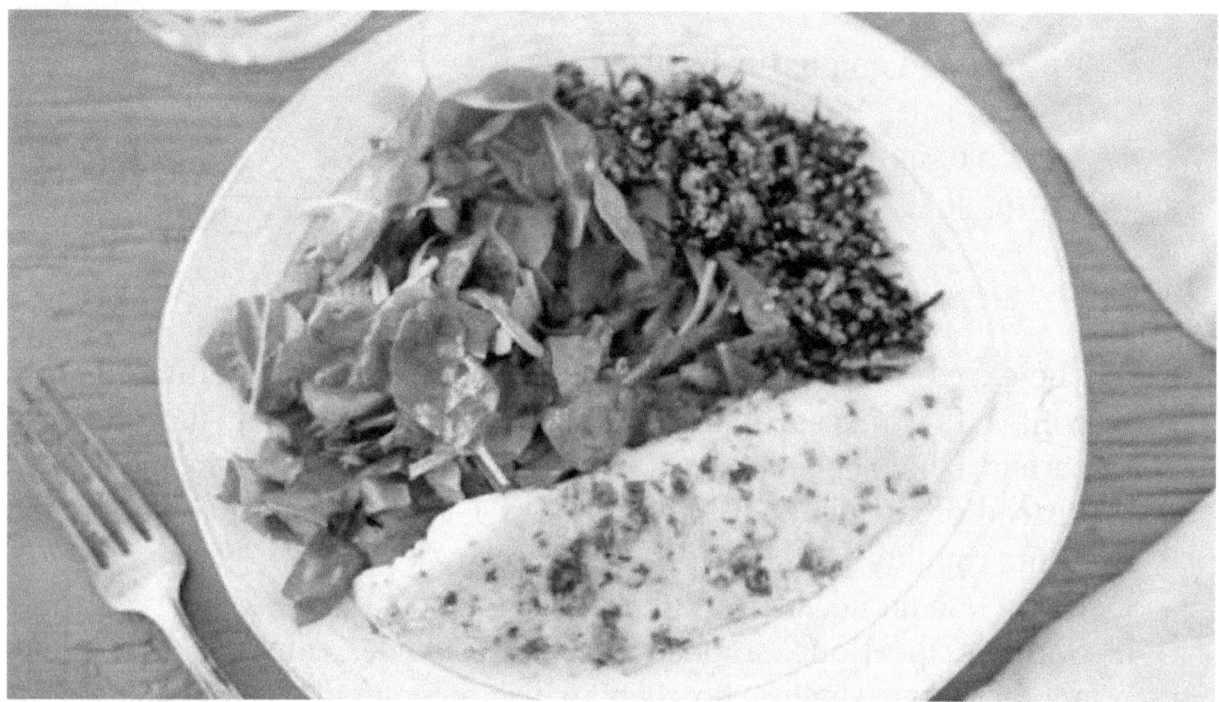

Ingredients

- 2 tbsps. of lemon juice
- 2 lbs. of tilapia fillets
- 1/2 cup of parmesan grated cheese
- 4 tbsps. of room temperature butter
- 3 tbsps. of mayonnaise
- 1 black pepper
- 3 tbsps. of green onions finely chopped
- 1/4 tsp. of seasoning salt
- 1/4 tsp. of dried basil
- pepper sauce (dash hot)

Directions

1. Set the oven to 350 degrees before you begin to cook.
2. Place the fillets in the prepared 13x9-inch baking dish or use jellyroll pan, arranging them in a single layer.
3. Fillets should not be stacked.
4. Brush the top with juice.
5. Put the butter, mayonnaise, onions, and spices in a bowl to make the cheese mixture.
6. Use a fork to mix well.
7. Fish in an oven set to the specified temperature for around 10 to 20 minutes will flake when done.
8. Let it spread out with the cheese mixture & bake until golden brown, approximately 5 minutes.
9. The time required for baking depends on the size of the fish.
10. Keep an eye on the fish so that it doesn't overcook.
11. Makes 4 servings.
12. Broil for 3 to 4 minutes, or until nearly done.
13. Add some cheese and broil for another 2 to 4 minutes, or until browned.

Conclusion

Intermittent fasting may be obtained in various ways, and there is no one-size-fits-all solution. Individuals will get the greatest results if they experiment with several styles to find which one best matches their lifestyle and tastes.

Fasting for long periods when the body is unprepared, regardless of intermittent fasting, might be harmful.

These diets may not be appropriate for everyone. These tactics may increase a person's negative connection with food if they are prone to disordered eating.

Before undertaking any fasting, anyone with health issues such as diabetes should see their doctor.

On non-fasting days, it's critical to consume a healthy and balanced meal for the greatest outcomes. To tailor an intermittent fasting regimen and prevent difficulties, a person might seek expert assistance if required.

It isn't for everyone, and it is only one of several preventative measures that may help you live longer. Quitting smoking, eating a low-salt, low-cholesterol diet, and participating in regular physical exercise are other strategies. These alternative disease prevention approaches have a lot more human scientific data than IF does. On the other hand, IF has a lot of potential as a health intervention, and it has the potential to go from alternative medicine to mainstream usage if science and practice are done properly. IF is making that shift, but more study is needed before making clinical assertions that can be used to reliably guide dietary recommendations and individual behavior.

To put it another way, researchers and scientists should be much more enthusiastic about the possibility of IF than the typical individual, who, as previously mentioned, can participate in more accessible (and proven) beneficial activities.

Intermittent fasting has been demonstrated to increase metabolism & fat burning while also conserving lean body mass, which may help you lose weight.

When used in combination with other diets, such as the keto, it may help speed up ketosis and prevent undesirable side effects like the keto flu.

Intermittent fasting may be a safe and successful weight management approach, while it may not perfect for everyone.

In conclusion, intermittent fasting is a feasible weight-loss strategy.

Its weight loss is mostly due to decreased calorie consumption, although some of its hormone-related benefits may also play a role.

Intermittent fasting isn't for everyone, but it may be quite helpful for certain individuals.

www.ingramcontent.com/pod-product-compliance
Lightning Source LLC
Chambersburg PA
CBHW081419080526
44589CB00016B/2597